D0790374

GET A JU
ON GOOD HEALTH
WITH
THE CORINNE T. NETZER FIBER COUNTER

If you want to increase fiber intake while not eating the same foods day after day, this book gives you the information you need. Discover a whole new world of surprising high-fiber alternatives to the old standby, oat bran:

- DRY-ROASTED, UNBLANCHED ALMONDS
  1 oz. = 3.9 grams

- *GREEN GIANT* FETTUCCINI PRIMAVERA
  1 pack = 6.0 grams

- PAPAYA
  1 medium = 5.5 grams

- *WONDER* LIGHT ITALIAN BREAD
  1 slice = 3.0 grams

- *PROGRESSO* MACARONI AND BEAN SOUP
  9.5 oz. = 6.5 grams

- RED RASPBERRIES
  ½ cup = 4.2 grams

THE CORINNE T. NETZER FIBER COUNTER

Corinne T. Netzer

A DELL BOOK

Published by
Dell Publishing
a division of
Bantam Doubleday Dell Publishing Group, Inc.
1540 Broadway
New York, New York 10036

ISBN: 0-440-21483-1

Printed in the United States of America

Published simultaneously in Canada

July 1994

10 9 8 7 6 5 4 3

OPM

THE
CORINNE T. NETZER
FIBER
COUNTER

Introduction

Fiber is the part of food that the human digestive system cannot absorb. Because it isn't a nutrient per se, fiber—or roughage, as it was called—used to be considered relatively unimportant. But the more scientists learned about the nature of fiber, the more they suggested it as a component of our daily diets. Today fiber is considered a vital element in maintaining our good health.

Fiber is divided into two categories: *water soluble* and *insoluble*. Although they act in different ways, both provide a laxative effect that helps the intestinal tract function. Since you are eliminating the waste of what you eat, the amount of indigestible residue in your diet makes a vast difference in the size, consistency, and frequency of your bowel movements. Fiber adds bulk by absorbing and holding on to water, thereby making the stool softer and easier to pass, as well as better able to stimulate the muscular action of the colon. It has long been acknowledged that intestinal ailments such as constipation and hemorrhoids can be avoided when stools are soft and passed often. And researchers now speculate that the risk of developing even more serious diseases may also be lessened with a high-fiber diet.

Studies indicate that people who traditionally live on very high fiber diets excrete often—as much as five to ten times the amount most Americans do—and they rarely suffer from diverticulosis or colon cancer, which is a leading killer in the United States. Speeding waste products through the system reduces our exposure to carcinogenic substances. In addition, fiber dilutes the concentration of these carcinogens and may even prevent their formation.

Although studies are not definitive as yet, it is also believed that a high-fiber diet may lower serum cholesterol, prevent or reverse hardening of the arteries, lower blood pressure, and aid in the prevention of breast cancer.

That's a lot of benefit from a substance we don't absorb, and fiber has still another advantage: because it isn't digested by saliva or stomach enzymes, it goes to the intestines "as is," providing a satisfying feeling of fullness—which is why many dieters experience great success with a high-fiber, low-fat regimen.

* * *

Until fairly recently, many people thought that fiber was just bran, and oat bran in particular, because so much had been written about it. Although oat bran does contain a good deal of fiber, it doesn't stand alone. There are as many kinds of bran as there are types of grain, and all are excellent sources of fiber. But fiber is found in a variety of foods besides bran and whole grains.

Every time you have a pea or a bean, every time you have a helping of broccoli or stir-fried vegetables, you are eating fiber. Fiber is present in *all* plant foods—in grains, fruits, vegetables, and legumes. Fortunately, these foods are also rich in vitamins and minerals, and they are among the most varied and delicious foods in the culinary world.

Instead of limiting yourself to bran and whole grains, this book enables you to choose from among a wide variety of foods. *The Corinne T. Netzer Fiber Counter* lets you know specifically which foods contain fiber—and how much. It tells you, for example, that there is more fiber in a half cup of cooked black beans or dried figs than in a half cup of many bran cereals or two slices of most whole-wheat breads.

The government has yet to establish strict guidelines for our daily fiber intake. However, nutritionists suggest that a healthy goal to aim for is an average intake of about twenty-five to thirty-five grams of fiber per day.

When on a high-fiber diet it is important to have plenty to drink. Inadequate liquid intake is a major reason for constipation. If you don't get enough water or other beverages, your body will absorb more water from the colon to meet its needs, making the stool difficult to pass.

Some people who are unaccustomed to a large quantity of fiber in their diets may initially experience some flatulence. Should this happen to you, cut back on your fiber intake and gradually build up to your goal.

* * *

Fiber should be eaten on a regular basis, and should replace much of the fats and refined carbohydrates in your diet. But it isn't an antidote for a diet rich in saturated fats and cholesterol. Don't have a bowl of bran for breakfast in addition to the bacon and eggs—have it *instead* of the bacon and eggs. Remember that fiber is essentially a preventative, not a cure; if you think you have any of the health problems mentioned above, you should seek your physician's help and advice.

The listings in the *Fiber Counter* are arranged alphabetically for easy reference. The fiber counts in this book are accompanied by a "c" (for *crude fiber*) or a "d" (for *dietary fiber*). Until recently, it was difficult for scientists to determine the fiber content of foods. For a long time a crude method of analysis was used, and the results of that analysis are known as crude fiber. However, this process failed to detect much of the actual fiber in food. An improved method of analysis was found, and the results from this process yield values known as dietary fiber. Unfortunately, dietary fiber listings are not yet available for all foods. I have given you the dietary fiber listings whenever they are available because they are a more accurate indication of the amount of fiber you are actually eating.

The data in this book has been compiled from information received from the United States Department of Agriculture and from individual food processors and purveyors. As we go to press, the information is the most complete and up-to-date available. When further data becomes available, I will be updating the *Fiber Counter*. In the meantime, good luck and good eating.

C.T.N.

Abbreviations & Symbols in This Book

c   . . . . . . crude fiber[1]

d   . . . . . . dietary fiber[1]

lb.   . . . . . . pounds

tsp.   . . . . . teaspoons(s)

tbsp. . . . . tablespoon(s)

tr.   . . . . . . trace

"   . . . . inch(es)

<   . . . . less than

(0)   . . . . . . may contain trace amounts

*   . . . . includes all varieties and
                 forms—without added
                 ingredients

[1] See page 4.

A

Abalone* 0
Abalone mushroom, see "Mushrooms, oyster"
Acerola, fresh:
untrimmed, 1 lb. . . . . 4.0 d
10 fruits, approximately 1.7 oz. untrimmed . . . . . . .5 d
trimmed, 1 cup . . . . 1.1 d
Acerola juice:
fresh, 6 fl. oz. . . . . .5 d
Acorn:
dried, 1 oz. . . . . 1.0 c
Acorn flour:
full fat, 1 oz. . . . . .8 c
Acorn squash:
raw, untrimmed, 1 lb. 5.2 d
raw, 1 medium, 4″ diameter, approximately
    1.2 lbs. untrimmed . . . . 6.5 d
baked, cubed, ½ cup . . . . 2.9 d
boiled, mashed, ½ cup . . . . 3.4 d
Adzuki bean confection, see "Yokan"
Adzuki beans, dry:
uncooked, 1 oz. . . . . 3.6 d
uncooked, ½ cup . . . . 12.4 d
boiled, ½ cup . . . . 2.3 c

Adzuki beans, canned:
(Eden), ½ cup . . . . 4.3 d
sweetened, ½ cup . . . . 2.3 c
Agar, see "Seaweed"
Alcoholic beverages, see specific listings
Alewife* 0
Alfalfa seeds, sprouted, raw:
1 oz. . . . . .7 d
½ cup . . . . .4 d
1 tbsp. . . . . .1 d
(Shaw's), 2 oz. . . . . <1.0 d
Alfalfa and dill seeds, sprouted:
raw *(Shaw's)*, 2 oz. . . . . 3.0 d
Alfalfa and radish seeds, sprouted:
raw *(Shaw's)*, 2 oz. . . . . <1.0 d
Alfredo sauce mix:
(Lawry's), 1 package . . . . .6 d
Allspice, ground:
1 oz. . . . . 6.1 d
1 tsp. . . . . .4 d
Almond butter:
plain or honey and cinnamon, 1 oz. . . . . 1.0 d
plain or honey and cinnamon, 1 tbsp. . . . . .5 d
Almond meal:
partially defatted, 1 oz. . . . . .7 c
Almond oil:
all varieties 0
Almond paste:
1 oz. . . . . 4.2 d
¼ cup firmly packed . . . . 8.5 d
1 tbsp. . . . . 2.1 d
Almonds, salted or unsalted:
(Beer Nuts), 1 oz. 3.0 d
dried, in shell, lb. 19.8 d
dried, shelled, unblanched:
  1 oz. . . . . 3.1 d

whole kernels, 1/2 cup . . . . 7.7 d
sliced, 1/2 cup . . . . 5.1 d
slivered, 1/2 cup . . . . 7.4 d
dried, shelled, blanched:
1 oz. . . . . 1.9 d
whole kernels, 1/2 cup . . . . 4.9 d
sliced, 1/2 cup . . . . 3.5 d
dry-roasted, unblanched, 1 oz. . . . . 3.9 d
dry-roasted, unblanched, whole kernels, 1/2 cup . 5.0 d
oil-roasted:
unblanched or blanched, 1 oz. . . . . 3.2 d
unblanched, whole kernels, 1/2 cup . . . . 8.9 d
blanched, whole kernels, 1/2 cup . . . . 8.0 d
toasted, 1 oz. . . . . 3.2 d
Amaranth:
raw, trimmed, 1/2 cup . . . . .1 c
boiled, drained, 1/2 cup . . . . .9 c
Amaranth, whole grain:
2 oz. . . . . 8.6 d
1/2 cup . . . . 14.9 d
Amaranth flakes:
(Arrowhead Mills), 1 oz. . . . . 3.0 d
Amaranth flour:
(Arrowhead Mills), 2 oz. . . . . 3.9 d
Amaranth seeds:
(Arrowhead Mills), 2 oz. . . . . 3.9 d
Amberjack* 0
Anasazi beans, dry:
uncooked (Arrowhead Mills), 2 oz. . . . . 12.1 d
Anchovies* 0
Anchovies, canned in oil* 0
Angel hair pasta, see "Pasta"
Anglerfish* 0
Anise seed:
1 oz. . . . . 4.1 d
1 tsp. . . . . .3 d

Apio root, see "Celeriac"

Apple:

raw, unpeeled:

  untrimmed, 1 lb. 11.3 d

  1 medium, 2¾″ diameter, approximately

    3 per lb. . . . . 3.7 d

  sliced, 1 cup . . . . 3.0 d

raw, peeled, 1 medium, 2¾″ diameter . . . . 2.4 d

raw, peeled, sliced, 1 cup . . . . 2.1 d

cooked, peeled, sliced, boiled, ½ cup . . . . 2.1 d

cooked, peeled, sliced, microwaved, ½ cup . . . . 2.4 d

Apple, canned:

for pie, see "Pie filling"

sweetened, sliced, drained, ½ cup . . . . 1.7 d

Apple, dehydrated, low moisture, sulfured:

uncooked, 2 oz. . . . . 7.0 d

uncooked, ½ cup . . . . 3.7 d

Apple, dried, sulfured:

uncooked, 2 oz. . . . . 4.9 d

uncooked, ½ cup . . . . 3.7 d

stewed, unsweetened, ½ cup . . . . 2.6 d

Apple, frozen:

unheated, 5 oz. . . . . 2.4 d

unsweetened, sliced, ½ cup . . . . 1.5 d

Apple butter:

spiced, 1 tbsp. . . . . .2 d

Apple cake, see "Cake" and "Cake, snack"

Apple cider, fresh, see "Apple juice"

Apple cobbler, see "Cobbler"

Apple crisp, frozen:

(*Pepperidge Farm* Classic), 4 oz. . . . . 1.0 d

Apple juice:

bottled, canned, or frozen and diluted, 6 fl. oz. . . .2 d

frozen concentrate, undiluted, 6-fl.-oz.

  container . . . . .8 d

Apple juice drink, 6 fl. oz. . . . . .2 d

Apple pie, see "Pie"
Apple pie spice:
(Tone's), 1 tsp. . . . . .7 d
Apple strudel:
2-oz. piece . . . . 1.2 d
Apple-cranberry juice drink:
bottled, 6 fl. oz. . . . . .2 d
Apple-raspberry juice drink:
bottled, 6 fl. oz. . . . . .2 d
Applesauce, in jars:
sweetened or unsweetened, 4 oz. . . . . 1.4 d
sweetened or unsweetened, ½ cup . . . . 1.5 d
Apricot, fresh:
untrimmed, 1 lb. . . . . 10.1 d
3 medium, approximately 12 per lb. . . . . 2.5 d
pitted, halves, ½ cup . . . . 1.9 d
Apricot, canned, in juice, syrup, or water:
unpeeled, 4 oz. . . . . 1.5 d
unpeeled, 3 halves and 1¾ tbsp. liquid . . . . 1.1 d
unpeeled, halves, ½ cup . . . . 1.6 d
Apricot, dried, sulfured:
uncooked:
2 oz. . . . . 5.1 d
10 halves, approximately 1.2 oz. . . . . 3.1 d
halves, ½ cup . . . . 5.9 d
cooked, unsweetened, halves, ½ cup . . . . 4.3 d
Apricot, frozen:
unheated, 5 oz. . . . . 2.4 d
sweetened, ½ cup . . . . 2.1 d
Apricot cobbler, see "Cobbler, frozen"
Apricot kernel oil:
all varieties 0
Apricot nectar:
canned or bottled, 6 fl. oz. . . . . 1.1 d
Aquavit:
all varieties 0

Arrowhead:
raw, 2⅝"-diameter corm. . . . . .1 c
boiled, 1"-diameter corm. . . . . .2 c
Arrowroot:
powder *(Tone's)*, 1 tsp. 0
Arrowroot flour:
2 oz. . . . . 2.0 d
½ cup . . . . 2.2 d
Artichoke,
globe or French:
raw, untrimmed, 1 lb. . . . . 9.8 d
raw, 1 medium, approximately 11.3 oz.
    untrimmed . . . . 6.9 d
boiled, drained:
    1 medium, 10.6 oz. . . . . 6.5 d
    hearts, 4 oz. . . . . 6.2 d
    hearts, ½ cup . . . . 4.5 d
Artichoke, canned, hearts:
with liquid *(Progresso)*, ½ cup . . . . 2.0 d
drained *(Progresso)*, ½ cup . . . . 3.0 d
marinated, with liquid *(Progresso)*, ½ cup . . . . . . 2.0 d
Artichoke, frozen:
hearts, 3 oz. . . . . 3.3 d
Artichoke, Jerusalem, see "Jerusalem
    artichoke"
Arugula, fresh, raw:
(Frieda's), 1 lb. . . . . 4.1 d
(Frieda's), 1 oz. . . . . .3 d
Asian pear, see "Pear, Asian"
Asparagus:
raw, untrimmed, 1 lb. . . . . 5.1 d
raw, 4 spears, approximately 3.8 oz. . . . . 1.2 d
boiled, 4 spears, ½" diameter base,
    approximately 2.1 oz. . . . . 1.3 d
boiled, drained, cuts, ½ cup . . . . 1.9 d

Asparagus, canned:

with liquid, 4 oz.	1.9 d
with liquid, cuts, ½ cup	2.1 d
drained, 4 oz.	1.8 d
drained, spears, ½ cup	1.9 d
spears, white or green, or cuts *(Green Giant)*, ½ cup	1.0 d

Asparagus, frozen:

unheated, 3.3 oz.	2.0 d
boiled, 4 spears, approximately 2.1 oz.	1.2 d
cuts *(Green Giant Harvest Fresh)*, ½ cup	2.0 d

Asparagus bean, see "Winged beans"

Asparagus pilaf:

frozen *(Green Giant Garden Right for Lunch)*, 9.5 oz.	3.0 d

Au jus gravy mix:

(Lawry's), dry, 1 packet	.1 c

Avocado:

California, 1 medium, 8 oz. untrimmed	10.2 d
Florida, 1 medium, 1 lb. untrimmed	17.9 d
all varieties, pulp, 1 oz.	1.7 d
all varieties, pureed, ½ cup	6.8 d

Avocado oil:

all varieties	0

B

Food and Measure	Fiber Grams

Babassu oil:
all varieties 0
Bacon, regular or Canadian style* 0
"Bacon," vegetarian:
.2-oz. strip .... .2 d
Bagel:
all varieties *(Thomas')*, 1 piece .... 1.0 d
plain, 2-oz. bagel .... 1.2 d
plain, onion, poppy seed, or sesame seed,
  1 bagel, 3½″ diameter, approximately 2½ oz. . 1.5 d
Bagel, frozen, 1 piece:
plain:
  (Lender's) .... 2.0 d
  (Lender's Bagel) .... 1.0 d
  (Lender's Big'N Crusty) .... 3.0 d
blueberry *(Lender's)* .... 2.0 d
cinnamon raisin *(Lender's/Lender's Big'N*
  Crusty). .... 2.0 d
egg *(Lender's)* .... 1.0 d
egg *(Lender's Big'N Crusty)* .... 2.0 d
oat *(Lender's)* .... 4.0 d
onion *(Lender's)* .... 2.0 d
poppy or sesame *(Lender's)* .... 2.0 d
rye or pumpernickel *(Lender's)* .... 2.0 d
soft *(Lender's* Original) .... 2.0 d

Baked beans, canned:

(Allens), 1/2 cup	5.0 d
(Campbell's Home Style), 4 oz.	13.0 d
(Grandma Brown's), 1/2 cup	7.8 d
(Grandma Brown's Saucepan), 1/2 cup	7.4 d
(Green Giant/Joan of Arc), 1/2 cup	6.0 d
barbecue *(Campbell's)*, 4 oz.	6.0 d
brown sugar and bacon *(Hanover)*, 1/2 cup	6.0 d
brown sugar and molasses *(Campbell's* Old Fashioned), 4 oz.	6.0 d
with frankfurters, 4 oz.	17.9 d
with frankfurters, 1/2 cup	8.8 d
with honey *(B&M* Brick Oven), 8 oz.	11.0 d
with honey, Boston *(Health Valley* Fat Free), 7.5 oz.	5.0 d
maple *(B&M* Brick Oven/*Friends)*, 8 oz.	11.0 d
with onions *(Bush's Best)*, 4 oz.	7.0 d
pea beans *(B&M* Brick Oven), 8 oz.	11.0 d

with pork:

1/2 cup	6.9 d
(Crest Top), 1/2 cup	5.0 d
(Hunt's), 4 oz.	8.0 d
(Wagon Master), 1/2 cup	5.0 d
pea beans, small *(Friends)*, 8 oz.	11.0 d
red kidney beans *(Friends)*, 8 oz.	11.0 d
and sweet sauce, 4 oz.	5.9 d
and sweet sauce, 1/2 cup	6.6 d
and tomato sauce, 4 oz.	5.5 d
and tomato sauce, 1/2 cup	6.0 d
tomato *(B&M* Brick Oven), 8 oz.	10.0 d
in tomato sauce *(Campbell's)*, 4 oz.	5.0 d
in tomato sauce *(Green Giant/Joan of Arc)*, 1/2 cup	5.0 d
red kidney beans *(B&M* Brick Oven), 8 oz.	11.0 d

vegetarian:

4 oz.	8.7 d

Baked beans, vegetarian *(cont.)*

½ cup . . . . 6.4 d

(B&M 50% Less Sodium), 8 oz. . . . . 11.0 d

(Bush's Deluxe), 4 oz. . . . . 6.0 d

honey baked, with miso *(Health Valley),*
7.5 oz. . . . . 5.4 d

in tomato sauce *(Campbell's),* 4 oz. . . . . 5.0 d

yellow eye *(B&M Brick Oven),* 8 oz. . . . . 11.0 d

Baking mix:

whole wheat *(Hain),* ⅓ cup . . . . 5.0 d

Baking powder:

(Davis), 1 tsp. 0

Baking soda:

(Tone's), 1 tsp. 0

Balsam pear, fresh:

leafy tips, boiled, drained, 4 oz. . . . . 2.1 d

leafy tips, boiled, drained, ½ cup . . . . .6 d

pods:

raw, untrimmed, 1 lb. . . . . 10.6 d

raw, 1 medium, 9⅜" long × 1½",
approximately 5.3 oz. . . . . 3.5 d

raw, ½" pieces, ½ cup . . . . 1.3 d

boiled, drained, ½" pieces, ½ cup . . . . 1.2 d

Bamboo shoots, fresh:

raw, trimmed, 4 oz. . . . . 2.5 d

raw, ½" slices, ½ cup . . . . 1.7 d

cooked, ½" slices, ½ cup . . . . 1.0 c

Bamboo shoots, canned:

(La Choy), ¼ cup . . . . <1.0 d

drained, 4 oz. . . . . 3.4 d

drained, ½ cup . . . . 2.0 d

Banana, fresh:

whole, 1 lb. . . . . 7.1 d

1 medium, 8¾" long, approximately 4 oz. . . . . . . 2.7 d

mashed, ½ cup . . . . 2.7 d

Banana, baking, see "Plantain"

Banana, dehydrated, powder:

1 oz.	2.1 d
1/4 cup	1.9 d
1 tbsp.	.5 d

Banana cake, see "Cake"

Banana chips:

1 oz.	2.2 d

Barbecue sauce:

1 oz.	.3 d
(Luzianne), 2 tbsp.	<1.0 d
(Lea & Perrins), 1 tbsp.	0
all varieties *(Hunt's)*, 1 tbsp.	<1.0 d
all varieties *(Ott's)*, 2 tbsp.	0
Oriental *(La Choy)*, 1 tbsp.	<.1 d
Oriental, stir-fry *(Lawry's)*, 1/4 cup	.2 c
sweet and sour *(Lawry's)*, 1/4 cup	.4 c

Barley:

uncooked:

2 oz.	9.8 d
1/2 cup	15.9 d
(Arrowhead Mills), 2 oz.	7.2 d
hulless *(Arrowhead Mills)*, 2 oz.	8.0 d

pearled:

uncooked, 2 oz.	8.9 d
uncooked, 1/2 cup	15.6 d
cooked, 1 cup	6.0 d

Barley flakes:

(Arrowhead Mills), 2 oz.	7.4 d

Barley flour:

(Arrowhead Mills), 2 oz.	7.2 d
Barracuda*	0

Basella, see "Vine spinach"

Basil, dried, ground:

1 oz.	5.0 d
1 tsp.	.2 d
Bass*	0

Bay leaf, dried, crumbled:

1 oz. . . . . 7.5 d

1 tsp. . . . . .2 d

Bean mix (see also specific bean listings),
  prepared:

(*Hunt's* Big John's Beans'n Fixin's), 4 oz. . . . . . . 6.0 d

Bean salad, canned:

three-bean (*Green Giant*), ½ cup . . . . 3.0 d

Bean sprouts, see "Sprouts" and specific
  bean listings

Beans, see specific listings

Beans, snap or string, see "Green beans"

Bearnaise sauce mix, dry:

.9-oz. packet . . . . .1 c

Beechnuts, dried:

shelled, 1 oz. . . . . 1.1 c

Beef* 0

Beef, corned or cured* 0

Beef, dried* 0

Beef chow mein, canned:

(*La Choy*), ¾ cup . . . . 2.0 d

(*La Choy* Bi-Pack), ¾ cup . . . . 1.0 d

Beef, pepper, entree, see "Steak, pepper"

Beef, roast, all cuts* 0

Beef gravy, canned:

¼ cup 0

Beef jerky:

all varieties 0

Beef luncheon meat:

all varieties, 4 oz. 0

Beef marinade seasoning mix:

(*Lawry's* Seasoning Blends), 1 package . . . . <.1 c

Beef stew seasoning mix, dry:

(*Lawry's* Seasoning Blends), 1 package . . . . 1.2 c

Beefalo* 0

Beer:

regular, 12 fl. oz. . . . . .7 d

light, 12 fl. oz. 0

Beerwurst:

all varieties, 4 oz. 0

Beet greens, fresh:

raw:

    untrimmed, 1 lb. . . . . 9.4 d

    1 leaf, approximately 2 oz. untrimmed . . . . . . 1.2 d

    1″ pieces, ½ cup . . . . .7 d

boiled, drained, 1″ pieces, ½ cup . . . . 2.1 d

Beets, fresh:

raw:

    without greens, untrimmed, 1 lb. . . . . 8.5 d

    2 medium, 2″ diameter, approximately 8.6 oz. . 4.6 d

    sliced, ½ cup . . . . 1.9 d

boiled, drained, 2 medium, 2″ diameter,

    approximately 3.5 oz. . . . . 1.7 d

boiled, drained, sliced, ½ cup . . . . 1.4 d

Beets, canned:

with liquid, 4 oz. . . . . 1.3 d

with liquid, ½ cup . . . . 1.4 d

drained, 4 oz. . . . . 2.1 d

drained, sliced, ½ cup . . . . 1.5 d

pickled, with liquid, sliced, ½ cup . . . . .7 c

Berliner:

pork and beef, 4 oz. 0

Berries, see specific listings

Berry punch:

bottled, 6 fl. oz. . . . . (0)

Berry-grape juice drink:

mixed berry *(Boku),* 8 fl. oz. 0

Biscuits:

(Wonder), 1 piece . . . . .6 d

breakfast, whole wheat country *(Awrey's 3″),*

    2 oz. . . . . 1.0 d

Biscuits *(cont.)*

round or square *(Awrey's 2")*, 1 oz.   0

sliced or unsliced *(Awrey's)*, 2 oz. . . . .   1.0 d

square *(Awrey's 3")*, 2 oz. . . . .   1.0 d

refrigerated:

   plain or buttermilk, 1-oz. piece . . . .   .4 d

   grain, mixed *(Roman Meal)*, 2 pieces . . . .   1.4 d

   honey-nut oat bran *(Roman Meal)*, 1 piece . . . . .   .9 d

   white *(Roman Meal)*, 1 piece   0

mix, dry, plain or buttermilk, 1 oz. . . . .   .7 d

mix, prepared, plain or buttermilk, 2-oz. piece . . .   1.0 d

Bitter melon, see "Balsam pear"

Black bean dishes, canned:

with tofu wieners *(Health Valley Tofu Fast
   Menu)*, 5 oz. . . . .   13.6 d

Western, with vegetables *(Health Valley Fast
   Menu Fat Free)*, 5 oz. . . . .   9.6 d

Black bean dishes, mix, prepared:

(Fantastic Instant), ½ cup . . . .   12.0 d

and rice *(Fantastic* Caribbean), 10 oz. . . . .   8.0 d

Black beans, dry (see also "Black turtle soup
   beans"):

uncooked:

   2 oz. . . . .   8.6 d

   ½ cup . . . .   14.7 d

   (Frieda's), 1 oz. . . . .   3.7 d

boiled, ½ cup . . . .   7.5 d

Black beans, canned:

(Eden No Salt Added), ½ cup . . . .   6.0 d

(Green Giant/Joan of Arc), ½ cup . . . .   6.0 d

(Progresso), 4 oz. . . . .   6.5 d

Black Forest torte, see "Cake"

Black turtle soup beans, dry:

uncooked:

   2 oz. . . . .   14.2 d

½ cup . . . . 22.9 d
(Arrowhead Mills), 2 oz. . . . . 11.3 d
boiled, ½ cup . . . . 4.9 d
Black turtle soup beans, canned:
(Hain), 4 oz. . . . . 6.0 d
Blackberries, fresh:
trimmed, 4 oz. . . . . 5.7 d
trimmed, ½ cup . . . . 3.6 d
Blackberries, canned:
in syrup, 4 oz. . . . . 3.9 d
in heavy syrup, ½ cup . . . . 4.4 d
Blackberries, frozen:
unsweetened, 5 oz. . . . . 7.1 d
unsweetened, ½ cup . . . . 3.8 d
Blackberry cobbler, see "Cobbler, frozen"
Blackeye peas, see "Cowpeas"
Blood sausage* 0
Bloody Mary cocktail mixer:
(Tabasco), 6 fl. oz. . . . . 1.0 d
extra spicy *(Tabasco)*, 6 fl. oz. . . . . 1.6 d
Blowfish* 0
Blueberries, fresh:
4 oz. . . . . 3.1 d
1 pint . . . . 10.9 d
½ cup . . . . 2.0 d
Blueberries, canned:
in syrup, 4 oz. . . . . 1.7 d
in heavy syrup, ½ cup . . . . 1.9 d
for pie, see "Pie filling"
Blueberries, frozen:
unsweetened, ½ cup . . . . 2.1 d
sweetened, ½ cup . . . . 2.4 d
Blueberry cobbler, see "Cobbler"
Blueberry-cranberry juice drink:
bottled, 6 fl. oz. . . . . (0)
Bluefish* 0

Boar, wild* 0
Bockwurst:
all varieties, 4 oz. 0
Bok choy, see "Cabbage, Chinese"
Bologna:
all meat or with cheese, 4 oz. 0
Bonito* 0
Borage:
raw, 1″ pieces, ½ cup . . . . .4 c
boiled, drained, 4 oz. . . . . 1.2 c
Boston cream pie, see "Pie, frozen"
Bouillon (see also "Soup"), dry:
all varieties *(Herb-Ox),* 1 cube, packet or tsp. . . . . . (0)
Bourbon:
all varieties 0
Boysenberries, fresh:
trimmed, 4 oz. . . . . 5.7 d
trimmed, ½ cup . . . . 3.6 d
Boysenberries, canned:
in syrup, 4 oz. . . . . 3.0 d
in syrup, ½ cup . . . . 3.3 d
Boysenberries, frozen:
unsweetened, 5 oz. . . . . 5.0 d
unsweetened, ½ cup . . . . 2.6 d
Brains* 0
Bran, see "Cereal" and specific listings
Brandy:
all varieties 0
Bratwurst:
all varieties, 4 oz. 0
Braunschweiger* 0
Brazil nuts, dried:
in shell, 1 lb. . . . . 13.5 d
shelled, 1 oz., 6 large or 8 medium kernels . . . . . 1.6 d
shelled, ½ cup . . . . 4.0 d

Bread:

apple-walnut swirl *(Pepperidge Farm)*, 1 slice . . . 2.0 d

(Arnold/Brownberry Bran'nola), 1 slice . . . . 3.0 d

bran:

  (Arnold Bakery Light Country), 1 slice . . . . 3.0 d

  (Brownberry Light Country), 1 slice . . . . 3.0 d

  honey *(Pepperidge Farm)*, 1 slice . . . . 1.0 d

  wheat, 1-oz. slice . . . . 2.4 d

  whole *(Brownberry* Natural), 1 slice . . . . 2.0 d

brown, see "Bread, brown"

brown and serve:

  Austrian wheat *(Bread du Jour)*, 1 oz. . . . . 1.2 d

  French *(Bread du Jour)*, 1 oz. . . . . .7 d

  French *(DiCarlo's* Parisian), 1 oz. . . . . .8 d

  French, petite *(Bread du Jour)*, 1 loaf . . . . 2.4 d

  grain, mixed, stick, soft *(Roman Meal)*,

    2.7 oz. . . . . 3.2 d

  grain, mixed, mini *(Roman Meal)*, 1/2 loaf . . . . . 2.4 d

cinnamon:

  chip *(Arnold)*, 1 slice . . . . <1.0 d

  raisin *(Wonder)*, 1 slice . . . . .9 d

  swirl *(Pepperidge Farm)*, 1 slice . . . . 2.0 d

corn bread, see "Bread, corn"

date nut bread, see "Bread, date nut"

French:

  1-oz. slice . . . . .8 d

  (Pepperidge Farm Fully Baked), 1 oz. 0

  (Wonder), 1 slice . . . . .7 d

  sliced or twin *(Pepperidge Farm)*, 1 oz. 0

  stick *(Savoni)*, 1 oz. . . . . 1.0 d

grain, mixed:

  (Roman Meal Round Top), 1 slice . . . . 1.2 d

  (Roman Meal Sandwich), 1 slice . . . . 1.0 d

  with oat bran *(Roman Meal)*, 1 slice . . . . 1.1 d

  nutty *(Arnold/Brownberry Bran'nola)*, 1 slice . . . 3.0 d

Bread, grain, mixed *(cont.)*

7, 1-oz. slice	2.0 d
7 *(Home Pride* Butter Top), 1 slice	1.2 d
7 *(Pepperidge Farm* Hearty), 1 slice	1.0 d
7 *(Pepperidge Farm* Light Style), 1 slice	2.0 d
7 *(Roman Meal),* 1 slice	1.2 d
7 *(Roman Meal* Light), 1 slice	2.6 d
with sunflower seeds *(Roman Meal* Sun Grain), 1 slice	1.4 d
12 *(Arnold* Natural), 1 slice	1.0 d
12 *(Brownberry* Natural), 1 slice	1.0 d
12 *(Roman Meal),* 1 slice	1.0 d
12 *(Roman Meal* Light), 1 slice	2.7 d
whole, 1-oz. slice	2.0 d
whole *(Roman Meal* 100%), 1 slice	2.2 d
health nut *(Brownberry* Natural), 1 slice	2.0 d
(Hollywood Special Formula Dark), 1 slice	.4 d
(Hollywood Special Formula Fitness Blend), 1 slice	1.0 d
(Hollywood Special Formula Light), 1 slice	.3 d
Italian:	
1-oz. slice	.9 d
(Arnold Bakery Light), 1 slice	2.0 d
(Brownberry Bakery Light), 1 slice	2.0 d
(Wonder Family), 1 slice	.7 d
(Wonder Light), 1 slice	3.0 d
oat:	
(Arnold/Brownberry Bran'nola Country), 1 slice	3.0 d
(Roman Meal), 1 slice	.8 d
crunchy *(Pepperidge Farm* Hearty), 1 slice	1.5 d
oat bran, 1 slice:	
1-oz. slice	1.3 d
(Roman Meal Light)	2.4 d
honey or honey nut *(Roman Meal)*	1.0 d

oatmeal:
  1-oz. slice . . . .   1.1 d
  (Arnold/Arnold Bakery), 1 slice . . . .   2.0 d
  (Brownberry Bakery Light), 1 slice . . . .   2.0 d
  (Brownberry Natural), 1 slice . . . .   1.0 d
  (Pepperidge Farm/Pepperidge Farm Light
    Style), 1 slice . . . .   1.0 d
  (Pepperidge Farm Thin), 1 slice . . . .   .5 d
  with bran *(Oatmeal Goodness* Light), 1 slice . . .   2.8 d
  with bran, sunflower or wheat *(Oatmeal
    Goodness)*, 1 slice . . . .   1.3 d
  raisin *(Arnold)*, 1 slice . . . .   2.0 d
  raisin *(Brownberry/Brownberry* Natural
    Sandwich), 1 slice . . . .   2.0 d
  soft *(Brownberry)*, 1 slice . . . .   2.0 d
  with wheat *(Oatmeal Goodness* Light), 1 slice .   2.8 d
orange raisin *(Brownberry)*, 1 slice . . . .   1.0 d
pan de aqua *(Arnold Augusto)*, 1 oz. . . . .   1.0 d
pita or pocket bread:
  oat bran *(Sahara)*, 1/2 piece . . . .   2.0 d
  wheat, whole, 1 piece, 6 1/2" diameter,
    approximately 2.3 oz. . . . .   4.8 d
  wheat, whole *(Sahara)*, 1 piece . . . .   5.0 d
  wheat, whole, mini *(Sahara)*, 1 piece . . . .   2.0 d
  white, 1 piece, 6 1/2" diameter, approximately
    2.1 oz. . . . .   2.3 d
  white *(Pepperidge Farm* Wholesome Choice),
    1 piece . . . .   2.0 d
  white, mini *(Pepperidge Farm* Wholesome
    Choice), 1 piece . . . .   1.0 d
  white *(Sahara)*, 1 mini or 1/2 regular . . . .   1.0 d
  white *(Sahara)*, 1/2 large . . . .   2.0 d
pumpernickel:
  1-oz. slice . . . .   1.7 d
  (Arnold), 1 slice . . . .   1.0 d
  (August Bros.), 1 slice . . . .   1.0 d

Bread, pumpernickel *(cont.)*

(Pepperidge Farm Family), 1 slice	2.0 d
(Pepperidge Farm Party), 4 slices	1.0 d
raisin, 1-oz. slice	1.2 d
raisin *(Arnold Sun-Maid)*, 1 slice	1.0 d

raisin cinnamon:

(Arnold), 1 slice	1.0 d
(Brownberry), 1 slice	1.0 d
swirl *(Pepperidge Farm)*, 1 slice	1.0 d
raisin walnut *(Brownberry)*, 1 slice	2.0 d

rye:

1-oz. slice	1.8 d
(Arnold Real Jewish Melba Thin), 1 slice	1.0 d
(Beefsteak Hearty/Soft), 1 slice	.8 d
(Beefsteak Mild), 1 slice	.9 d
(Pepperidge Farm Party), 4 slices	1.0 d
caraway *(Brownberry* Natural), 1 slice	1.0 d
caraway or Dijon *(Arnold* Real Jewish), 1 slice	1.0 d
Dijon *(Pepperidge Farm)*, 1 slice	1.0 d
dill *(Arnold)*, 1 slice	1.0 d
dill *(Brownberry* Natural), 2 slices	1.0 d
onion *(August Bros.)*, 1 slice	1.0 d
onion *(Beefsteak)*, 1 slice	.8 d
pumpernickel *(Brownberry* Natural), 1 slice	1.0 d
seeded *(Pepperidge Farm* Family), 1 slice	2.0 d
seeded or seedless *(August Bros.)*, 1 slice	1.0 d
seeded or seedless *(Levy's* Real Jewish), 1 slice	1.0 d
seedless *(Arnold* Real Jewish), 1 slice	1.0 d
seedless *(Brownberry* Natural), 2 slices	1.0 d
seedless *(Pepperidge Farm* Family), 1 slice	2.0 d
soft *(Arnold Bakery* Light), 1 slice	2.0 d
soft *(Brownberry Bakery* Light), 1 slice	2.0 d
soft, seeded or unseeded *(Arnold Bakery)*, 1 slice	1.0 d
rye and pumpernickel *(August Bros.)*, 1 slice	1.0 d

sandwich, dark *(Brownberry* Natural), 1 slice . . . .   2.0 d
sourdough:
  (Francisco), 1 slice . . . .   1.0 d
  (Roman Meal Light), 1 slice . . . .   2.6 d
  (Wonder Light), 1 slice . . . .   3.0 d
  whole grain *(Roman Meal)*, 1 slice . . . .   1.3 d
  whole grain *(Roman Meal* Light), 1 slice . . . . .   2.7 d
sunflower and bran *(Monk's)*, 1 oz. . . . .   2.0 d
Vienna, 1-oz. slice . . . .   .8 d
Vienna *(Pepperidge Farm* Light Style), 1 slice . . .   1.0 d
wheat:
  1-oz. slice . . . .   1.2 d
  (Arnold Brick Oven), 1 slice . . . .   2.0 d
  (Arnold Natural), 1 slice . . . .   2.0 d
  (Beefsteak Hearty), 1 slice . . . .   1.4 d
  (Brownberry Hearth), 1 slice . . . .   2.0 d
  (Brownberry Natural), 1 slice . . . .   2.0 d
  (Fresh & Natural), 1 slice . . . .   1.6 d
  (Home Pride ButterTop), 1 slice . . . .   1.4 d
  (Home Pride Honey ButterTop), 1 slice . . . . . .   1.8 d
  (Home Pride Light), 1 slice . . . .   2.4 d
  (Pepperidge Farm 1½ lb.), 1 slice . . . .   2.0 d
  (Pepperidge Farm Light Style), 1 slice . . . .   1.0 d
  (Pepperidge Farm Family 2 lb.), 1 slice . . . . . .   2.0 d
  (Pepperidge Farm Very Thin), 2 slices   0
  (Roman Meal Light), 1 slice . . . .   2.6 d
  (Thomas' Light), 1 slice . . . .   2.0 d
  (Wonder Country Style/Golden), 1 slice . . . . . .   1.0 d
  (Wonder Family), 1 slice . . . .   .9 d
  (Wonder Light), 1 slice . . . .   2.0 d
  apple honey *(Brownberry)*, 1 slice . . . .   2.0 d
  cracked, 1-oz. slice . . . .   1.5 d
  cracked *(Pepperidge Farm* Thin), 2 slices . . . .   1.0 d
  cracked *(Roman Meal)*, 1 slice . . . .   2.2 d
  cracked *(Wonder)*, 1 slice . . . .   .8 d

Bread, wheat *(cont.)*

   dark or hearty *(Arnold/Brownberry Bran'nola),*
     1 slice . . . . 3.0 d
   golden *(Arnold Bakery* Light), 1 slice . . . . 2.0 d
   golden *(Brownberry* Light), 1 slice . . . . 2.0 d
   hearty *(Roman Meal* Light), 1 slice . . . . 2.5 d
   honey wheatberry *(Arnold),* 1 slice . . . . 2.0 d
   honey wheatberry *(Roman Meal),* 1 slice . . . . . 1.0 d
   reduced calorie, 1-oz. piece . . . . 3.2 d
   sesame *(Pepperidge Farm* Hearty), 1 slice . . . . 1.5 d
   soft *(Brownberry),* 1 slice . . . . 1.0 d
   sprouted *(Pepperidge Farm),* 2 slices . . . . 2.0 d
   wheatberry *(Roman Meal* Light), 1 slice . . . . . . 2.5 d
  wheat, whole:
   1-oz. slice . . . . 2.0 d
   (Arnold Brick Oven Light 100%), 1 slice . . . . . 3.0 d
   (Arnold Stone Ground 100%), 1 slice . . . . 2.0 d
   (Pepperidge Farm Thin), 2 slices . . . . 2.0 d
   (Roman Meal Light 100%), 1 slice . . . . 2.4 d
   (Roman Meal 100%), 1 slice . . . . 2.1 d
   (Wonder Stoneground 100%), 1 slice . . . . 2.2 d
   regular or soft *(Wonder* 100%), 1 slice . . . . . . 1.7 d
  wheatberry, 1-oz. slice . . . . 1.2 d
  white:
   1-oz. slice . . . . .7 d
   (Arnold Bakery Light Premium), 1 slice . . . . . . 2.0 d
   (Arnold Brick Oven), 1 slice . . . . 1.0 d
   (Arnold Brick Oven Light), 1 slice . . . . 2.0 d
   (Arnold Brick Oven Thin), 1 slice . . . . <1.0 d
   (Arnold Country), 1 slice . . . . 1.0 d
   (Beefsteak Robust), 1 slice . . . . .7 d
   (Brownberry Country), 1 slice . . . . 1.0 d
   (Brownberry Natural), 1 slice . . . . <1.0 d
   (Home Pride ButterTop), 1 slice . . . . 1.4 d
   (Home Pride Light), 1 slice . . . . 2.4 d
   (Pepperidge Farm Country), 2 slices . . . . 2.0 d

(Pepperidge Farm Large Family/Thin/Very
  Thin), 1 slice 0
(Roman Meal Light), 1 slice . . . . 2.6 d
(Wonder), 1 slice . . . . .7 d
(Wonder Light), 1 slice . . . . 2.0 d
with buttermilk *(Wonder)*, 1 slice . . . . .7 d
extra fiber *(Arnold Brick Oven)*, 1 slice . . . . . . 2.0 d
reduced calorie, 1-oz. slice . . . . 2.6 d
sandwich *(Brownberry)*, 1 slice . . . . <1.0 d
sandwich *(Pepperidge Farm)*, 2 slices 0
soft *(Brownberry)*, 1 slice . . . . 1.0 d
toasting *(Pepperidge Farm)*, 1 slice . . . . 1.0 d
Bread, brown, canned:
½″ slice, approximately 1.6 oz. . . . . 2.1 d
regular or raisin *(B&M/Friends)*, ½″ slice . . . . . . 2.0 d
Bread, corn, mix:
dry, 8.5-oz. package 15.4
prepared, ⅙ of square 8″ pan, approximately
  2.1 oz. 1.4
Bread, date nut:
(Thomas'), 1-oz. slice . . . . 1.0 d
Bread crumbs:
dry, plain, 1 oz. . . . . 1.2 d
dry, plain, ½ cup . . . . 2.3 d
plain or Italian *(Arnold)*, ½ oz. . . . . <1.0 d
seasoned *(Contadina)*, 1 rounded tbsp. . . . . .1 d
soft, white, 1 cup . . . . 1.0 d
Bread dough:
frozen, white *(Rich's)*, 2 slices . . . . .8 d
refrigerated *(Roman Meal)*, 1 oz. . . . . .6 d
refrigerated, country oatmeal or cracked wheat
  and honey *(Hearty Grains)*, 1″ slice . . . . 1.0 d
Bread shell, Italian:
(Boboli, 6″), 1 piece . . . . 2.0 d
(Boboli, 12″), 1 piece . . . . 8.0 d
Bread stuffing, see "Stuffing"

Breadfruit:

½ cup . . . . 5.4 d

¼ small, approximately 3.4 oz. . . . . 4.7 d

Breadfruit seeds, shelled:

raw, South American cultivar, 1 oz. . . . . .5 c

boiled, Pacific area cultivar, 1 oz. . . . . .5 c

roasted, South American cultivar, 1 oz. . . . . .6 c

Breadnut tree seeds:

dried, 1 oz. . . . . 4.2 d

Breadsticks:

cheddar or onion *(Pepperidge Farm* Thin),

½ oz. . . . . 1.0 d

refrigerated, soft *(Roman Meal),* 1 piece . . . . .8 d

Broad beans, immature:

raw:

   untrimmed, 1 lb. 18.5 d

   10 beans, approximately 2.8 oz. untrimmed . . . 3.4 d

   ½ cup . . . . 2.3 d

boiled, drained, 4 oz. 2.2 c

Broad beans, mature, dry:

raw, 2 oz. . . . . 14.2 d

raw, ½ cup . . . . 18.8 d

boiled, ½ cup . . . . 4.6 d

Broad beans, mature, canned:

(Progresso Fava Beans), ½ cup . . . . 12.0 d

Broccoli, fresh:

raw:

   untrimmed, 1 lb. 8.3 d

   1 spear, approximately 8.7 oz. . . . . 4.5 d

   chopped, ½ cup . . . . 1.3 d

boiled, drained, 1 spear, approximately 6.3 oz. . . 5.2 d

boiled, drained, chopped, ½ cup . . . . 2.3 d

Broccoli, frozen:

spears *(Green Giant* Select), ½ cup . . . . 3.0 d

spears or chopped, 10-oz. package . . . . 8.5 d

spears or chopped, boiled, drained, ½ cup . . . . . 2.8 d

spears or cuts *(Green Giant Harvest Fresh),*
    ½ cup . . . . 2.0 d
spears, cuts, or chopped *(Stilwell),* ½ cup . . . . . 2.0 d
cuts *(Green Giant Polybag),* ½ cup . . . . 4.0 d
in butter sauce, cut *(Green Giant One Serving),*
    4.5 oz. . . . . 3.0 d
in butter sauce, spears *(Green Giant),* ½ cup . . . 2.0 d
in cheese sauce:
    (Birds Eye), ½ cup . . . . 2.0 d
    (Green Giant), ½ cup . . . . 2.0 d
    cut *(Green Giant One Serving),* 5 oz. . . . . 2.0 d
Broccoli combinations, frozen:
carrots and rotini, in cheese sauce *(Green Giant*
    One Serving), 5.5 oz. . . . . 3.0 d
and cauliflower *(Frosty Acres Swiss Mix),* 3 oz. . 1.0 c
and cauliflower medley *(Green Giant Valley*
    Combinations), ½ cup . . . . 3.0 d
cauliflower and carrots:
    (Green Giant One Serving), 4 oz. . . . . 3.0 d
    in butter sauce *(Green Giant),* ½ cup . . . . 3.0 d
    in cheese sauce *(Birds Eye),* ½ cup . . . . 2.0 d
    in cheese sauce *(Green Giant One Serving),*
       5 oz. . . . . 2.0 d
    in cheese sauce *(Green Giant),* ½ cup . . . . . . 2.0 d
fanfare *(Green Giant Valley Combinations),*
    ½ cup . . . . 3.0 d
and red peppers *(Green Giant Select),* ½ cup . . . 2.0 d
Broth, see "Soup"
Brown gravy, in jars:
(Heinz HomeStyle), 2 oz. or ¼ cup . . . . .3 d
(La Choy), ½ tsp. . . . . <1.0 d
Brown gravy mix:
dry *(Lawry's),* 1 package . . . . .2 c
prepared *(Pillsbury),* ¼ cup 0
prepared *(Spatini),* 1 cup . . . . .1 c

Brownies:

1 small square, 1¾″ × ¾″, approximately 1 oz. . .	.7 d
1 large square, 2¾″ × ⅞″, approximately 2 oz. . . .	1.3 d
(Tastykake), 1 piece	5.0 d
all varieties (Hostess Brownie Bites), 5 pieces . . .	1.8 d
fudge nut (Awrey's Sheet Cake), 1.2 oz.	1.0 d
fudge nut, iced (Awrey's Sheet Cake), 2.5 oz.	1.0 d

Browning sauce:

(Gravymaster), 1 tsp.	tr.c

Brussels sprouts, fresh:

raw, untrimmed, 1 lb.	17.2 d
raw, ½ cup	1.8 d
boiled, drained, 1 sprout, approximately ¾ oz. . .	.9 d
boiled, drained, ½ cup	3.4 d

Brussels sprouts, frozen:

unheated, 3.3 oz.	3.6 d
boiled, drained, ½ cup	1.4 d
(Birds Eye), 3.3 oz.	3.0 d
in butter sauce (Green Giant), ½ cup	4.0 d

Buckwheat:

2 oz.	5.7 d
½ cup	8.5 d

Buckwheat flour:

whole groat, 2 oz.	5.7 d
whole groat, ½ cup	6.0 d
(Arrowhead Mills), 2 oz.	7.1 d

Buckwheat groats:

brown or white (Arrowhead Mills), 2 oz.	7.1 d

Buffalo fish* 0

Bulgur (see also "Tabbouleh mix"):

uncooked, 2 oz.	10.4 d
uncooked, ½ cup	12.8 d
cooked, ½ cup	4.1 d

Buns, see "Rolls"

Buns, sweet (see also "Rolls, sweet"):
honey:
   glazed, 1 oz. . . . . .6 d
   glazed, 1 small, 4" × 3", approximately 2.3 oz. . 1.4 d
   glazed, 1 large, 5" × 3½", approximately 3 oz. . 1.8 d
   glazed *(Tastykake)*, 1 piece . . . . 4.0 d
   iced *(Tastykake)*, 1 piece . . . . 1.0 d
frozen, cinnamon *(Rich's Ever Fresh)*, 1 piece . . . 1.9 d
frozen, honey *(Rich's Ever Fresh)*, 1 piece . . . . . . 1.0 d
Burbot* 0
Burdock root:
raw:
   untrimmed, 1 lb. . . . . 11.2 d
   1 medium, approximately 7.3 oz. . . . . 5.1 d
   pieces, ½ cup . . . . 1.9 d
boiled, drained, 1 medium root . . . . 3.0 d
boiled, drained, 1" pieces, ½ cup . . . . 1.1 d
Burrito dinner mix:
(Tio Sancho Dinner Kit):
   seasoning, 3.25 oz. . . . . 5.5 c
   1 tortilla . . . . .1 c
Burrito seasoning mix, dry:
(Lawry's Seasoning Blends), 1 package . . . . .9 c
(Old El Paso), ⅛ package . . . . 1.0 d
Butter:
all varieties, salted or unsalted 0
Butter beans, see "Lima beans"
Butter flavor seasoning:
all flavors *(McCormick/Shilling Best O' Butter)*,
   ½ tsp. 0
Butter oil:
plain or flavored 0
Butterbur, fresh:
raw, ½ cup . . . . .6 c
raw, 1 stalk, approximately .2 oz. . . . . .1 c
boiled, drained, 4 oz. .9 c

Butterbur, canned:

3 stalks, approximately 1.6 oz.	.4 c
chopped, 1/2 cup	.6 c

Butterfish* 0

Buttermilk:

fluid or dry 0

Butternut squash, fresh:

raw, untrimmed, 1 lb.	5.7 d
raw, cubed, 1/2 cup	1.1 d
fresh, baked, cubed, 1/2 cup	2.9 d

Butternut squash, frozen:

unheated, 4 oz.	1.5 d
boiled, drained, 4 oz. or 1/2 cup mashed	1.0 c

Butternuts, dried:

in shell, 1 lb.	5.8 d
shelled, 1 oz.	1.3 d

Butterscotch, see "Candy"

Butterscotch baking chips:

(*Nestlé* Toll House Morsels), 1 oz. .... (0)

C

Food and Measure	Fiber Grams

Cabbage:
raw:
  untrimmed, 1 lb. . . . . 8.4 d
  1 head, 5¾″ diameter, approximately 2½ lbs.
    untrimmed . . . . 20.9 d
  shredded, ½ cup .8 d
boiled, drained, ½ head . . . . 17.7 d
boiled, drained, shredded, ½ cup . . . . 2.1 d
Cabbage, Chinese:
bok choy:
  raw, untrimmed, 1 lb. . . . . 4.0 d
  raw, shredded, ½ cup . . . . .4 d
  boiled, drained, shredded, ½ cup . . . . 1.4 d
pe-tsai:
  raw, whole, untrimmed, 1 lb. . . . . 4.2 d
  raw, shredded, ½ cup . . . . .4 d
  boiled, drained, shredded, ½ cup . . . . 1.0 d
Cabbage, red:
raw, untrimmed, 1 lb. . . . . 7.3 d
raw, shredded, ½ cup . . . . .7 d
boiled, drained, 1 leaf, approximately ¾ oz. . . . . . .4 d
boiled, drained, shredded, ½ cup . . . . 1.5 d

Cabbage, savoy:

raw, whole, untrimmed, 1 lb. . . . . 11.2 d

raw, shredded, 1/2 cup . . . . 1.1 d

boiled, drained, shredded, 1/2 cup . . . . .5 c

Cactus pear, see "Prickly pear"

Cajun seasoning:

(Tone's), 1 tsp. . . . . .5 d

Cake:

angel food, 1/12 of 9" cake, approximately 1 oz. . . . .4 d

apple streusel *(Awrey's),* 2" square 0

banana, iced *(Awrey's),* 2" square 0

Black Forest torte *(Awrey's),* 1/14 cake . . . . 1.0 d

Boston cream, see "Pie, frozen"

carrot, supreme, iced *(Awrey's),* 2" square 0

carrot, 3-layer, iced *(Awrey's),* 1/12 cake . . . . 1.0 d

cheesecake, 1/6 of 17-oz. cake, approximately

   2.8 oz. . . . . 1.7 d

chocolate:

  with chocolate frosting, 1/8 of 18-oz. cake,

    approximately 2 1/4 oz. . . . . 1.8 d

  double, iced *(Awrey's),* 2" square . . . . 1.0 d

  double, 2-layer *(Awrey's),* 1/12 cake . . . . 1.0 d

  double, 3-layer *(Awrey's),* 1/12 cake . . . . 2.0 d

  double, torte *(Awrey's),* 1/14 cake . . . . 2.0 d

  fudge, chocolate frosted, 1/8 of 18-oz. cake,

    approximately 2 1/4 oz. . . . . 1.8 d

  German, iced *(Awrey's),* 2" square 0

  German, 3-layer *(Awrey's),* 1/12 cake . . . . 1.0 d

  milk, yellow, 2-layer *(Awrey's),* 1/12 cake 0

  white iced, 2-layer *(Awrey's),* 1/12 cake . . . . . . 1.0 d

coconut, butter cream *(Awrey's),* 2" square 0

coconut, yellow, 3-layer *(Awrey's),* 1/12 cake 0

coffee cake:

  caramel nut or long John *(Awrey's),* 1/12 cake 0

  cheese, 1/6 of 1-lb. cake, approximately

    2.7 oz. . . . . .9 d

cinnamon, with crumb topping, 1/9 of 20-oz.
cake, approximately 2.2 oz. . . . .   2.1 d
creme-filled, chocolate frosted, 1/6 of 19-oz.
cake, approximately 3.2 oz. . . . .   1.8 d
fruit, 1/8 of 14-oz. cake, approximately
1.75 oz. . . . .   1.3 d
devil's food, chocolate frosted, 1/8 of 18-oz.
cake, approximately 2 1/4 oz. . . . .   1.8 d
devil's food, iced (Awrey's), 2" square . . . .   1.0 d
fruitcake, 1.5-oz. piece . . . .   1.5 d
lemon, 2-layer or 3-layer (Awrey's), 1/12 cake   0
Neapolitan torte (Awrey's), 1/14 cake   0
orange, frosty, iced (Awrey's), 2" square   0
orange, three-layer, iced (Awrey's), 1/12 cake   0
peanut butter torte (Awrey's), 1/14 cake . . . .   1.0 d
pistachio torte (Awrey's), 1/14 cake . . . .   1.0 d
pound, 1/10 of 10.6-oz. cake, approximately
1.1 oz. . . . .   .3 d
pound, golden (Awrey's), 1/12 cake   0
raisin spice, iced (Awrey's), 2" square   0
raspberry nut (Awrey's), 1/16 cake   0
sponge (Awrey's), 2" square   0
strawberry supreme torte (Awrey's), 1/12 cake . . . .   1.0 d
walnut torte (Awrey's), 1/14 cake   0
yellow, chocolate frosting, 3.5 oz. . . . .   1.8 d
yellow, iced (Awrey's), 2" square   0
Cake, snack:
apple pastry pocket (Tastykake), 1 piece . . . .   1.0 d
apple spice:
(Hostess Light), 1 piece . . . .   .5 d
(Hostess Twinkies), 1 piece . . . .   .5 d
(Tastykake Creamie), 1 piece . . . .   1.0 d
brownie, see "Brownies"
butterscotch (Tastykake Krimpets), 1 piece   0
cheese pastry pocket (Tastykake), 1 piece . . . . .   1.0 d
cherry pastry (Tastykake), 1 piece . . . .   1.0 d

Cake, snack *(cont.)*

chocolate:

(Hostess Choco Bliss), 1 piece	1.2 d
(Hostess Choco-Diles), 1 piece	1.5 d
(Hostess Ding Dongs), 1 piece	1.0 d
(Hostess Grizzly Chomps), 1 piece	.8 d
(Hostess Ho Hos), 1 piece	.6 d
(Hostess Suzy Q's), 1 piece	2.0 d
(Tastykake Creamie), 1 piece	1.0 d
(Tastykake Junior), 1 piece	4.0 d
(Tastykake Kandy Kakes), 1 piece	1.0 d

coconut:

(Tastykake Junior), 1 piece	3.0 d
(Tastykake Kandy Kake), 1 piece	1.0 d
covered *(Hostess Sno Balls)*, 1 piece	1.0 d

coffee cake:

(Tastykake Koffee Kake Junior), 1 piece	1.0 d
cinnamon crumb *(Hostess 97% Fat Free)*, 1 piece	.4 d
cream filled *(Tastykake Koffee Kake)*, 1 piece	0
crumb *(Hostess)*, 1 piece	.7 d

cupcake:

butter cream, cream filled *(Tastykake)*, 1 piece .	1.0 d
chocolate *(Hostess)*, 1 piece	.9 d
chocolate *(Tastykake)*, 1 piece	1.0 d
chocolate *(Tastykake Royale)*, 1 piece	2.0 d
chocolate, cream filled *(Tastykake)*, 1 piece . . .	1.0 d
chocolate, cream filled *(Tastykake Tasty Too)*, 1 piece	1.0 d
chocolate, creme filled *(Hostess Lights)*, 1 piece	.9 d
creme *(Tastykake Kreme Kup)*, 1 piece	1.0 d
orange *(Hostess)*, 1 piece	.5 d
vanilla, cream filled *(Tastykake Tasty Too)*, 1 piece	1.0 d

date-nut pastry *(Awrey's)*, 1.6 oz. piece . . . . | 1.0 d |

donut, see "Donuts"

golden, cream filled *(Hostess Twinkies)*, 1 piece . . .5 d

golden, cream filled *(Hostess Twinkies* Lights),
  1 piece . . . . .4 d

(Hostess Dessert Cup), 1 piece . . . . .4 d

(Hostess Tiger Tails), 1 piece . . . . 1.3 d

jelly *(Tastykake Krimpets)*, 1 piece . . . . 1.0 d

lemon or orange *(Tastykake* Junior), 1 piece . . . . 1.0 d

peanut butter *(Tastykake* Kandy Kakes), 1 piece . 1.0 d

strawberry *(Tastykake Krimpet)*, 1 piece 0

strawberry filled *(Hostess Twinkies Fruit N
  Creme)*, 1.5-oz. piece . . . . .5 d

vanilla *(Hostess Grizzly Chomps)*, 1 piece . . . . .8 d

vanilla *(Tastykake* Creamie), 1 piece . . . . 1.0 d

Cake mix, prepared:

cheesecake, no-bake type, 3.5 oz. . . . . 1.9 d

gingerbread, 1/9 of square 8″ cake,
  approximately 2.6 oz. . . . . 2.4 d

lemon, orange, pineapple supreme, lemon-
  poppyseed, or orange-walnut *(Simply
  Splendid)*, 3 oz. . . . . 1.0 d

Calabash gourd, see "White-flowered gourd"

Calves liver* 0

Candy:

(Baby Ruth), 1 oz. . . . . .8 d

(Bar None), 1 oz. . . . . .9 d

(Butterfinger), 1 oz. . . . . .8 d

butterscotch, 1 oz. 0

candy corn, 1 oz. 0

caramel, plain, 1 oz. . . . . .3 d

caramel, chocolate flavor roll, 1 oz. . . . . .2 d

carob, 1 oz. . . . . 1.8 d

chocolate:

  milk, 1 oz. . . . . 1.0 d

  milk, with almonds, 1 oz. . . . . 1.8 d

  milk, with crisps *(Nestlé Crunch)*, 1 oz. . . . . . .7 d

Candy, chocolate *(cont.)*

milk, with fruit and nuts *(Chunky)*, 1 oz.	1.4 d
milk, with peanuts *(Mr. Goodbar)*, 1 oz.	1.2 d
milk, with rice cereal, 1 oz.	.7 d
white, with almonds *(Alpine White)*, 1 oz.	1.5 d
semisweet, 1 oz.	1.7 d
sweet, 1 oz.	1.6 d
sweet *(Hershey's Special Dark)*, 1 oz.	1.6 d
coconut, chocolate coated *(Mounds)*, 1 oz.	.9 d
coconut, toasted *(Andes Thins)*, 8 pieces	0
cookie bar, caramel *(Twix)*, 1 oz.	.5 d
cookie bar, peanut butter *(Twix)*, 1 oz.	.9 d
cough drops *(Hall's Tablets)*, 1 piece	0
fondant	0
fondant, chocolate coated, 1 oz.	.3 d
fruit chews *(Starburst)*, 2.07 oz.	0
fruit flavored, all flavors *(Skittles)*, 2.3 oz.	0
fudge, homemade:	
chocolate, 1 oz.	.2 d
chocolate, with nuts, 1 oz.	.4 d
vanilla, 1 oz.	0
vanilla, with nuts, 1 oz.	.2 d
grape *(Heide Cool Grape)*	0
gum, chewing, all flavors, 1 oz.	0
gumdrops, 1 oz.	0
hard, all flavors, 1 oz.	0
jellied and gummed, all varieties, 1 oz.	0
(Kit Kat), 1 oz.	.3 d
licorice, 1 oz.	0
lollipops, all flavors, 1 oz.	0
(M&M's Plain or Peanut), 1 oz.	.9 d
(Mars), 1 oz.	.6 d
marshmallow, 1 oz.	(0)
(Milky Way), 1 oz.	.5 d
mint, all flavors, 1 oz.	0
nougat, 1 oz.	0

(Oh Henry!), 1 oz.	1.0 d
(100 Grand), 1 oz.	(0)
peanut bar, 1 oz.	.9 d
peanut brittle, 1 oz.	.6 d
peanuts, chocolate coated, 1 oz.	2.9 d
peanuts, chocolate coated *(Goobers)*, 1⅜ oz.	3.0 d
popcorn, caramel, see "Popcorn"	
raisins, chocolate coated, 1 oz.	1.2 d
(Reese's Pieces/Reese's Peanut Butter Cups)*, 1 oz.	1.2 d
rock candy, 1 oz.	0
(Rolo), 1 oz.	.2 d
sesame crunch, 1 oz.	2.2 d
(Snickers), 1 oz.	.9 d
sour balls, 1 oz.	0
taffy, all flavors, 1 oz.	0
(3 Musketeers), 1 oz.	.5 d
toffee, 1 oz.	0
(Whatchamacallit), 1 oz.	.9 d
Cane syrup:	
1 tbsp.	0
Cannellini, see "Kidney beans"	
Canola oil:	
all varieties	0
Cantaloupe, fresh:	
untrimmed, 1 lb.	1.9 d
½ of 5"-diameter melon, approximately 1.1 lbs. untrimmed	2.1 d
pulp, 1 oz.	.2 d
pulp, cubed, ½ cup	.6 d
Capers:	
1 tablespoon	0
Capon*	0
Caponata, see "Eggplant appetizer"	
Cappicola ham:	
all varieties, 4 oz.	0

Cappuccino, bottled:

hot, all varieties *(Maxwell House)*, 6 fl. oz. 0

iced, all varieties *(Chock o'ccino)*, 8 fl. oz. 0

iced, all varieties *(Maxwell House Cappio)*,

  8 fl. oz. 0

Captain D's, 1 serving:

dinner[1]:

  chicken, with salad . . . . 3.9 d

  fish, baked, with salad . . . . 4.4 d

  orange roughy, with salad . . . . 3.9 d

  shrimp, with slaw . . . . 3.9 d

side dishes:

  cole slaw, 4 oz. . . . . 1.9 d

  crackers, 4 pieces . . . .   .2 d

  cracklin's, 1 oz. 0

  dinner salad, without dressing . . . . 1.4 d

  green beans, seasoned, 4 oz. . . . . 1.4 d

  hush puppy, 1 piece . . . .   .1 d

  rice, 4 oz. . . . . 1.1 d

  white beans, 4 oz. 3.0 d

dressings, blue cheese, French, Italian, or

  ranch, 1 packet 0

sauces, cocktail, sweet and sour, or tartar, side

  portion. 0

desserts:

  carrot cake, cheesecake, or chocolate cake,

    1 slice 0

  lemon pie, 1 slice 0

  pecan pie, 1 slice . . . . 4.4 d

Carambola, fresh:

1 medium, approximately 4.7 oz. . . . . 3.4 d

cubed, ½ cup . . . . 1.9 d

Caramel topping:

(Smucker's), 2 tbsp. 0

[1] Includes rice, green beans, and breadstick.

Caraway seeds:
1 tsp. . . . . .8 d
Cardamom:
ground *(Tone's)*, 1 tsp. . . . . .2 d
seed *(Spice Islands)*, 1 tsp. . . . . .2 c
Cardoon, raw:
untrimmed, 1 lb. 3.6 d
trimmed, shredded, ½ cup . . . . 1.4 d
Carissa:
1 medium, approximately .8 oz. . . . . .2 c
sliced, ½ cup . . . . .7 c
Carob drink mix:
powder, 3 tsp. . . . . .2 c
Carob flour:
2 oz. . . . . 22.6 d
½ cup . . . . 20.1 d
1 tbsp. . . . . 3.2 d
Carp* 0
Carrot, fresh:
raw:
   without greens, untrimmed, 1 lb. . . . . 12.1 d
   1 medium, 7½″ long, approximately 2.8 oz.
      untrimmed . . . . 2.2 d
   trimmed, shredded, ½ cup . . . . 1.7 d
boiled, 1 medium, approximately 1.6 oz. . . . . . . 1.5 d
boiled, drained, sliced, ½ cup . . . . 2.6 d
Carrot, canned:
with liquid, 4 oz. . . . . 1.0 d
drained, 4 oz. . . . . 1.7 d
drained or with liquid, sliced, ½ cup . . . . 1.1 d
Carrot, frozen:
unheated, 3.3 oz. 3.0 d
boiled, drained, sliced, ½ cup . . . . 2.6 d
whole, baby *(Green Giant Harvest Fresh/*
   Select), ½ cup . . . . 2.0 d

Carrot juice:

canned or bottled, 6 fl. oz. . . . .   1.5 d

Casaba:

untrimmed, 1 lb. . . . .   2.2 d

2″ slice, ¹⁄₁₀ of 7³⁄₄″ melon, approximately

  8.6 oz. untrimmed . . . .   1.3 d

trimmed, 1 oz. . . . .   .2 d

trimmed, cubed, ½ cup . . . .   .7 d

Cashew butter:

1 oz. . . . .   .6 d

1 tbsp. . . . .   .3 d

Cashews:

(Beer Nuts), 1 oz. . . . .   1.0 d

dry-roasted, 1 oz., approximately 18 medium . . . .   .9 d

dry-roasted, whole or halves, ½ cup . . . .   2.1 d

oil-roasted, 1 oz., approximately 18 medium . . . .   1.1 d

oil-roasted, whole or halves, 1 cup . . . .   4.9 d

Cassava, raw:

untrimmed, 1 lb. . . . .   .5 d

trimmed, 1 oz. . . . .   <.1 d

Catfish*   0

Catfish entree, Cajun:

frozen *(Gorton's),* 1 piece   0

Catjang:

boiled, ½ cup . . . .   1.4 c

Catsup:

1 oz. . . . .   .5 d

1 packet . . . .   .1 d

1 tbsp. . . . .   .2 d

(Hunt's/Hunt's No Salt Added), 1 tbsp. . . . .   <1.0 d

Cauliflower, fresh:

raw:

  untrimmed, 1 lb. . . . .   4.4 d

  3 flowerets, approximately 5 oz. untrimmed . . .   1.4 d

  trimmed, 1″ pieces, ½ cup . . . .   1.3 d boiled, drained, 3 flowerets, approximately

    1.9 oz. . . . . 1.5 d

boiled, drained, 1″ pieces, ½ cup . . . . 1.7 d

Cauliflower, frozen:

unheated, 3.3 oz. . . . . 2.2 d

boiled, drained, 1″ pieces, ½ cup . . . . 2.0 d

cuts *(Green Giant),* ½ cup . . . . 2.0 d

breaded *(Stilwell),* 13 pieces . . . . 3.0 d

frozen, in cheese sauce:

  (Birds Eye), 5 oz. 1.0 d

  (Green Giant), ½ cup . . . . 2.0 d

  (Green Giant One Serving), 5.5 oz. . . . . 2.0 d

Cavatelli:

frozen *(Celentano),* 3.2 oz. . . . . 9.0 d

Caviar* 0

Cayenne, see "Pepper"

Ceci, see "Chickpeas"

Celeriac, fresh, raw:

untrimmed, 1 lb. . . . . 7.0 d

trimmed, 4 oz. . . . . 2.1 d

trimmed, ½ cup . . . . 1.4 d

Celery, fresh:

raw:

  without greens, untrimmed, 1 lb. . . . . 6.9 d

  1 stalk, 7½″, approximately 1.6 oz.

    untrimmed . . . . .7 d

  trimmed, diced, ½ cup . . . . 1.0 d

boiled, drained, diced, ½ cup . . . . 1.2 d

Celery flakes:

dried *(Tone's),* 1 tsp. . . . . .3 d

Celery root, see "Celeriac"

Celery salt:

(Tone's), 1 tsp. . . . . .2 d

Celery seeds, dried:

1 oz. . . . . 3.3 d

1 tsp. . . . . .2 d

Cellophane noodles, see "Noodles, Chinese"
Celtus:
raw, trimmed, 1 oz. . . . . .1 c
Cereal, ready-to-eat, dry:
bran (see also "oat bran," below):
  (All Bran), 1 oz. 9.0 d
  (Arrowhead Mills Bran Flakes), 1 oz. . . . . 4.1 d
  (Bran Buds), 1 oz. . . . . 11.0 d
  (Bran Chex), 1 oz. . . . . 4.0 d
  (Kellogg's Bran Flakes), 1 oz. . . . . 5.0 d
  (Kellogg's Fiberwise), 1 oz. . . . . 5.0 d
  (Nabisco 100% Bran), 1 oz. . . . . 10.0 d
  (Post Bran Flakes), 1 oz. . . . . 5.0 d
  extra fiber *(All Bran),* 1 oz. . . . . 14.0 d
  with fruit *(Kellogg's Fruitful Bran),* 1 oz. with
    .4 oz. fruit . . . . 5.0 d
bran, with raisins:
  (Erewhon Raisin Bran), 1 oz. . . . . 3.0 d
  (General Mills Raisin Nut Bran), 1 oz. . . . . 2.5 d
  (Kellogg's Raisin Bran), 1 oz. with .4 oz.
    raisins . . . . 5.0 d
  (Malt-O-Meal Raisin Bran), 1.4 oz. . . . . 5.0 d
  (Nutri· Grain), 1 oz. with .4 oz. raisins . . . . . . 5.0 d
  (Post Raisin Bran), 1.4 oz. . . . . 6.0 d
  (Skinner's Raisin Bran), 1 oz. . . . . 4.0 d
  (Total Raisin Bran), 1.5 oz. . . . . 4.0 d
corn:
  (Arrowhead Mills Flakes), 1 oz. . . . . 2.8 d
  (Corn Pops), 1 oz. 1.0 d
  (Honeycomb), 1 oz. . . . . tr. d
  (Kellogg's Corn Flakes/Frosted Flakes), 1 oz. . 1.0 d
  (Malt-O-Meal), 1 oz. . . . . 1.0 d
  (Nut & Honey Crunch), 1 oz. 0
  (Nutri· Grain), 1 oz. 3.0 d
  (Post Toasties), 1 oz. . . . . tr. d
  apple *(Arrowhead Mills* Apple Corns), 1 oz. . . . 3.0 d

golden *(Health Valley Fruit Lites)*, 1 oz. . . . . .8 d
maple *(Arrowhead Mills Maple Corns)*, 1 oz. . . . 3.0 d
puffed *(Arrowhead Mills)*, .5 oz. . . . . .4 d
sugar frosted *(Malt-O-Meal)*, 1 oz. . . . . 1.0 d
granola:
   (C.W. Post Hearty), 1 oz. . . . . tr. d
   all varieties *(Health Valley* Fat Free), 1 oz. . . . . 2.5 d
   with bran *(Erewhon #9)*, 1 oz. . . . . 4.0 d
   maple nut *(Arrowhead Mills)*, 1 oz. . . . . 11.9 d
kamut flakes *(Erewhon)*, 1 oz. . . . . 4.0 d
kashi, puffed *(Kashi)*, .75 oz. . . . . 2.0 d
millet, puffed *(Arrowhead Mills)*, .5 oz. . . . . .5 d
mixed grain and natural style:
   (Almond Delight), 1 oz. . . . . 1.0 d
   (Apple Jacks), 1 oz. 1.0 d
   (Arrowhead Mills Arrowhead Crunch), 1 oz. . . . 3.5 d
   (Basic 4), 1.3 oz. . . . . 2.0 d
   (Cinnamon Toast Crunch), 1 oz. . . . . 1.0 d
   (Clusters), 1 oz. . . . . 2.0 d
   (Crispix), 1 oz. . . . . 1.0 d
   (Crunchy Nut Oh!s), 1 oz. . . . . .9 d
   (Double Dip Crunch), 1 oz. 0
   (Erewhon Aztec), 1 oz. . . . . 1.0 d
   (Erewhon Right Start), 1 oz. . . . . 5.0 d
   (Erewhon Super-O's), 1 oz. . . . . 4.0 d
   (Fiber One), 1 oz. . . . . 13.0 d
   (Froot Loops), 1 oz. 1.0 d
   (Fruit & Frosted O's), 1 oz. . . . . 1.0 d
   (Grape Nuts/Grape Nuts Flakes), 1 oz. . . . . . . 3.0 d
   (Honey Graham Oh!s), 1 oz. . . . . .7 d
   (Just Right), 1 oz. . . . . 2.0 d
   (Multi Grain Cheerios), 1 oz. . . . . 2.0 d
   (Product 19), 1 oz. . . . . 1.0 d
   (Quaker 100% Natural), 1 oz. . . . . 2.0 d
   (Special K), 1 oz. . . . . 1.0 d
   (Sunflakes Multi-Grain), 1 oz. . . . . 3.0 d

Cereal, ready-to-eat, mixed grain and natural style *(cont.)*

(Total), 1 oz.	2.0 d
(Uncle Sam), 1 oz.	7.0 d
all varieties *(Health Valley* Fiber Flakes), 1 oz.	5.0 d
all varieties *(Health Valley O's* Fat Free), 1 oz.	5.0 d
with almonds *(Honey Bunches of Oats),* 1 oz.	1.0 d
almond raisin *(Nutri· Grain),* 1 oz. with .4 oz. nuts and fruit	3.0 d
with apple *(Erewhon Apple Stroodles),* 1 oz.	3.0 d
apple and almond *(Kellogg's Mueslix Golden Crunch),* 1 oz.	3.0 d
apple raisin *(Apple Raisin Crisp),* 1 oz. with .3 oz. fruit	3.0 d
with banana *(Erewhon Banana-O's),* 1 oz.	2.0 d
with bananas and Hawaiian fruit *(Sprouts 7),* 1 oz.	4.3 d
cinnamon *(Kellogg's* Mini Buns), 1 oz.	1.0 d
cinnamon and raisin *(Nature Valley),* 1 oz.	1.0 d
dates, raisins, and walnuts *(Fruit & Fibre),* 1.25 oz.	5.0 d
with fiber nuggets *(Just Right),* 1 oz.	2.0 d
with fruit and nuts *(Kellogg's Mueslix Crispy Blend),* 1.5 oz.	3.0 d
fruit and nut *(Nature Valley),* 1 oz.	1.0 d
honey-roasted *(Honey Bunches of Oats),* 1 oz.	1.0 d
peaches, raisins, and almonds *(Fruit & Fibre),* 1.25 oz.	5.0 d
pecan, double *(Post Great Grains),* 1.25 oz.	3.0 d
pineapple, banana, and coconut *(Fruit & Fibre),* 1.25 oz.	5.0 d
plain or raisin *(Heartland),* 1 oz.	2.0 d
with raisins *(Erewhon Right Start),* 1 oz.	5.0 d
raisin *(Grape Nuts),* 1 oz.	2.0 d
with raisins *(Sprouts 7),* 1 oz.	4.7 d

raisins, dates, and nuts *(Just Right)*, 1 oz.
with .3 oz. fruit and nuts . . . . 2.0 d
raisin, date, and pecan *(Post Great Grains)*,
1.25 oz. . . . . 3.0 d
muesli *(Master Choice)*, 2 oz. . . . . 5.0 d
oat:
  (Alpha-Bits), 1 oz. . . . . 1.0 d
  (Cheerios), 1 oz. . . . . 2.0 d
  (Cinnamon Life), 1 oz. . . . . 2.5 d
  (General Mills Oatmeal Crisp), 1 oz. . . . . 1.0 d
  (Honey Bunches of Oats), 1 oz. . . . . 2.0 d
  (Honey Nut Cheerios), 1 oz. . . . . 1.5 d
  (Life), 1 oz. . . . . 2.5 d
  (Nut & Honey Crunch O's), 1 oz. . . . . 1.0 d
  (Toasty O's), 1 oz. . . . . 2.0 d
  with almonds *(Honey Bunches of Oats)*, 1 oz. . 2.0 d
  apple cinnamon *(Cheerios)*, 1 oz. . . . . 1.5 d
  apple and cinnamon *(Toasty O's)*, 1 oz. . . . . . 1.0 d
  honey bran *(Kellogg's Oatbake)*, 1 oz. . . . . . . 3.0 d
  honey and nut *(Toasty O's)* . . . . 2.0 d
  marshmallow *(Alpha-Bits)*, 1 oz. . . . . 1.0 d
  with raisins *(General Mills Oatmeal Raisin
    Crisp)*, 1.2 oz. . . . . 1.5 d
  raisin nut *(Kellogg's Oatbake)*, 1 oz. . . . . 3.0 d
  toasted *(Nature Valley)*, 1 oz. . . . . 1.0 d
  toasted, rings *(Skinner's)*, 1 oz. . . . . 3.0 d
oat bran:
  (Arrowhead Mills Flakes), 1 oz. . . . . 3.4 d
  (Common Sense), 1 oz. . . . . 3.0 d
  (Cracklin' Oat Bran), 1 oz. . . . . 4.0 d
  (Post Oat Flakes), 1 oz. . . . . 2.0 d
  (Skinner's), 1 oz. 4.0 d
  with raisins *(Common Sense)*, 1 oz. with
    .3 oz. raisins . . . . 3.0 d
oatmeal, toasted or honey nut *(Quaker)*, 1 oz. . . . 2.0 d

rice:
  (Erewhon Poppets), 1 oz. . . . .   1.0 d
  (Frosted Krispies), 1 oz.   0
  (Rice Krispies), 1 oz.   0
  chocolate (Cocoa Krispies), 1 oz.   0
rice, brown:
  (Health Valley Fruit Lites), .5 oz. . . . . .5 d
  crispy (Erewhon/Erewhon Low Sodium), 1 oz. .   1.0 d
  crispy (Kellogg's Kenmei), 1 oz. . . . .   1.0 d
rice, puffed:
  (Arrowhead Mills), .5 oz. . . . . .4 d
  (Malt-O-Meal), .5 oz.   0
  (Quaker), .5 oz. . . . . .2 d
wheat:
  (Kellogg's Smacks), 1 oz. . . . .   1.0 d
  (Malt-O-Meal Sugar Puffs), 1 oz. . . . .   1.0 d
  (Nutri· Grain), 1 oz. . . . .   3.0 d
  (Total), 1 oz. . . . .   3.0 d
  (Wheat Chex), 1 oz. . . . .   2.0 d
  (Wheaties), 1 oz. . . . .   3.0 d
  (Wheaties Honey Gold), 1 oz. . . . .   1.0 d
  apple-cinnamon filled (Kellogg's Apple
     Cinnamon Squares), 1 oz. . . . .   2.0 d
  blueberry filled (Kellogg's Blueberry Squares),
     1 oz. . . . .   3.0 d
  flakes (Erewhon), 1 oz. . . . .   3.0 d
  with fruit (Erewhon Fruit'n Wheat), 1 oz. . . . . .   3.0 d
  golden (Health Valley Fruit Lites), 1 oz. . . . . . .   1.0 d
  with raisins (Crispy Wheat 'N Raisins), 1 oz. . . .   2.0 d
  raisin filled (Kellogg's Raisin Squares), 1 oz. . . .   2.0 d
  strawberry filled (Kellogg's Strawberry
     Squares), 1 oz. . . . .   3.0 d
wheat, puffed (Arrowhead Mills), .5 oz. . . . . .9 d
wheat, puffed (Malt-O-Meal), .5 oz. . . . .   1.0 d
wheat, shredded:
  (Kellogg's Frosted Mini Wheats), 1 oz. . . . .   3.0 d

(Nabisco), 1 piece . . . .   3.0 d
(Nutri· Grain), 1 oz. . . . .   4.0 d
(S.W. Graham), 1 oz. . . . .   3.0 d
bran (Nabisco Shredded Wheat'n Bran), 1 oz. .   4.0 d
cinnamon (S.W. Graham), 1 oz. . . . .   2.0 d
mini (Nabisco Spoon Size), 1 oz. . . . .   3.0 d
whole grain (Kellogg's), 1 oz. . . . .   4.0 d
wheat bran, see "bran," above
Cereal, cooking[1] (see also specific grains):
bran (H-O Brand Super Bran), 1/3 cup . . . .   8.0 d
farina, see "wheat," below
granola (H-O Brand), 1/2 cup . . . .   5.0 d
mixed grain:
   (Arrowhead Mills Seven Grain), 1 oz. . . . .   4.0 d
   (Erewhon Organic Barley Plus), 1 oz. . . . .   1.0 d
   (Roman Meal Original), 1 oz. . . . .   4.9 d
   apple cinnamon (Roman Meal), 1.2 oz. . . . . . .   6.4 d
   with oats (Roman Meal Original), 1.2 oz. . . . . .   4.8 d
oat bran:
   (Arrowhead Mills), 1 oz. . . . .   7.9 d
   (Roman Meal), 1 oz. . . . .   4.7 d
   with toasted wheat germ (Erewhon Oat Bran),
      1 oz. . . . .   3.0 d
oatmeal and oats:
   (Arrowhead Mills Instant), 1 oz. . . . .   4.3 d
   (H-O Brand Quick/Instant Box), 1/3 cup . . . . . .   3.0 d
   (H-O Brand Instant), 1 packet . . . .   3.0 d
   (Instant Quaker), 1 packet . . . .   2.8 d
   apple cinnamon (Instant Quaker), 1 packet . . . .   3.0 d
   apple cinnamon (Quaker Oat Cups), 5.5 oz.
      container . . . .   2.9 d
   apple, date, and almond (Arrowhead Mills
      Instant), 1 oz. . . . .   3.7 d
   apple spice (Arrowhead Mills Instant), 1 oz. . . .   3.4 d

[1] Uncooked, except as noted.

Cereal, cooking, oatmeal and oats *(cont.)*

bananas and cream *(Instant Quaker)*,
1 packet . . . .   2.0 d

blueberries and cream *(Instant Quaker)*,
1 packet . . . .   1.9 d

cinnamon, raisin, and almond *(Arrowhead
Mills* Instant), 1 oz. . . . .   4.3 d

with fiber *(H-O Brand* Instant), 1 packet . . . . .   3.0 d

with fiber *(H-O Brand* Instant Box), ⅓ cup . . . .   3.0 d

with fiber, apple or raisin, and bran *(H-O
Brand* Instant), 1 packet . . . .   3.0 d

maple brown sugar *(H-O Brand* Instant),
1 packet . . . .   3.0 d

maple brown sugar *(Instant Quaker)*, 1 packet .   2.9 d

with oat bran *(Erewhon* Instant), 1.25 oz. . . . . .   4.0 d

peaches and cream *(Instant Quaker)*,
1 packet . . . .   2.3 d

raisin, date, and walnut *(Erewhon* Instant),
1.2 oz. . . . .   3.0 d

strawberries and cream *(Instant Quaker)*,
1 packet . . . .   2.2 d

sweet'n mellow *(H-O Brand* Instant), 1 packet .   3.0 d

with wheat, date, raisin, and almond *(Roman
Meal)*, 1.3 oz. . . . .   3.0 d

with wheat, honey, coconut, almond *(Roman
Meal)*, 1.3 oz. . . . .   2.7 d

rice, brown *(Arrowhead Mills Rice & Shine)*,
¼ cup . . . .   1.6 d

rye, cream of *(Roman Meal)*, 1.3 oz. . . . .   5.4 d

wheat:

(Arrowhead Mills Bear Mush) . . . .   1.3 d

(Malt-O-Meal) . . . .   1.0 d

(Wheatena) . . . .   4.0 d

bulgur *(Arrowhead Mills)*, 2 oz. . . . .   5.4 d

chocolate *(Malt-O-Meal)* . . . .   1.0 d

cracked *(Arrowhead Mills)*, 2 oz. . . . .   2.3 d

farina, cream *(H-O Brand)*, 3 tbsp. . . . . 3.0 d
maple and brown sugar *(Malt-O-Meal)* . . . . . . 1.0 d
with oat bran *(Malt-O-Meal* Plus 40%),
  1.3 oz. . . . . 3.0 d
Cereal bar, see "Granola and cereal bars"
Cereal beverage, see "Coffee substitute"
Cervelat:
beef or pork, 4 oz. 0
Chablis wine 0
Champagne, all varieties 0
Chard, see "Swiss chard"
Chardonnay wine 0
Chayote, raw:
untrimmed, 1 lb. 13.5 d
1 medium, approximately 7.2 oz. untrimmed . 6.1 d
1" pieces, ½ cup . . . . 2.0 d
boiled, drained, 1" pieces, ½ cup . . . . .5 c
Cheddarwurst:
all varieties, 4 oz. 0
Cheese* 0
Cheese dip:
(Chi-Chi's Fiesta), 1 oz. 0
nacho, jalapeño *(Price's)*, 1 oz. . . . . .1 d
Cheese food* 0
Cheese sauce mix:
dry, 1 oz. . . . . .3 d
Cheese spread:
all varieties, 1 oz. 0
Cheese sticks, frozen:
cheddar, breaded *(Stilwell)*, 1 piece . . . . 1.0 d
mozzarella, battered *(Stilwell)*, 1 piece . . . . 1.0 d
Cheesecake, see "Cake" and "Cake mix"
Cherimoya:
1 medium, approximately 1.9 lb. . . . . 13.1 d
Cherry, maraschino:
in jars, with liquid, 1 oz. . . . . .1 c

Cherry cobbler, see "Cobbler, frozen"
Cherry juice drink:
bottled, 6 fl. oz. . . . . (0)
Cherry pastry, see "Cake, snack"
Cherry-grape juice drink:
(Boku), 8 fl. oz. 0
Cherries, fresh:
sour, red:
   with pits, 4 oz. . . . . 1.4 d
   with pits, ½ cup . . . . .6 d
   pitted, 4 oz. . . . . 1.4 d
   pitted, ½ cup . . . . .9 d
sweet:
   with pits, 4 oz. . . . . 2.4 d
   with pits, ½ cup . . . . 1.7 d
   10 medium, approximately 2.6 oz. . . . . 1.6 d
   pitted, 4 oz. . . . . 2.6 d
   pitted, ½ cup . . . . 1.7 d
Cherries, canned:
sour, pitted, in syrup, 4 oz. . . . . .9 d
sour, pitted, in heavy syrup, ½ cup . . . . 1.0 d
sweet, pitted, in syrup, 4 oz. . . . . .8 d
sweet, pitted, in heavy syrup, ½ cup . . . . .9 d
for pie, see "Pie filling"
Cherries, frozen:
sour, red, unsweetened, 4 oz. . . . . 1.4 d
sour, red, unsweetened, ½ cup . . . . .9 d
sweet, sweetened, 4 oz. . . . . 1.1 d
sweet, sweetened, ½ cup . . . . 1.3 d
Chervil, dried:
1 oz. . . . . 3.2 d
1 tsp. . . . . .1 d
Chestnuts, Chinese, shelled:
raw, 1 oz. . . . . .5 c
dried, 1 oz. . . . . .8 c

boiled or steamed, 1 oz. . . . . .3 c
roasted, 1 oz. . . . . .5 c
Chestnuts, European:
raw, in shell, 1 lb. . . . . 27.2 d
raw, shelled, with peel, ½ cup, approximately
  6 kernels . . . . 5.9 d
dried, peeled, 1 oz. . . . . 1.4 c
boiled, 1 oz. . . . . .2 c
roasted:
  in shell, 1 lb. . . . . 36.9 d
  shelled, 1 oz. . . . . 3.7 d
  ½ cup, approximately 8 kernels . . . . 5.5 d
Chestnuts, Japanese:
raw, 1 oz. . . . . .3 c
dried, 1 oz. . . . . .6 c
boiled or steamed, 1 oz. . . . . .1 c
roasted, 1 oz. . . . . .3 c
Chewing gum, see "Candy"
Chick-fil-A, 1 serving:
sandwiches:
  chicken . . . . .7 c
  chicken, char grilled . . . . .1 c
  chicken, char grilled, deluxe . . . . .1 c
  chicken deluxe . . . . .7 c
  chicken salad . . . . 1.4 c
  Chick-N-Q . . . . 1.4 c
chicken dishes:
  garden salad, char grilled . . . . 3.7 c
  Grilled'n Lites, 2 skewers . . . . tr. c
  Nuggets, 8-pack . . . . .6 c
  salad plate . . . . 4.1 c
side dishes:
  carrot and raisin salad, cup . . . . 1.0 c
  chicken soup, breast of, hearty, cup . . . . .7 c
  coleslaw, cup . . . . 1.1 c
  potato salad, cup .7 c

Chick-fil-A, side dishes *(cont.)*
  tossed salad . . . .   2.1 c
  tossed salad, with blue cheese or ranch
    dressing . . . .   2.1 c
  tossed salad, with honey French dressing . . . .   2.4 c
  tossed salad, with lite Italian or Thousand
    Island dressing . . . .   2.2 c
  tossed salad, with lite ranch dressing . . . .   2.1 c
desserts:
  cheesecake . . . .   .1 c
  cheesecake, with blueberry topping . . . .   .4 c
  cheesecake, with strawberry topping . . . .   .5 c
  fudge brownie, with nuts . . . .   .3 c
  Icedream, small cup . . . .   .3 c
  lemon pie . . . .   .3 c
lemonade, small . . . .   .1 c
Chicken*   0
Chicken batter seasoning, Cajun:
(Tone's), 1 tsp. . . . .   .1 d
Chicken bologna:
all varieties, 4 oz.   0
Chicken chow mein, see "Chicken entree"
Chicken entree, canned or packaged:
chow mein:
  (La Choy), ¾ cup . . . .   2.0 d
  (La Choy Bi-Pack),* ¾ cup . . . .   1.0 d
  (La Choy Dinner),* ½ package . . . .   2.0 d
sweet and sour:
  (La Choy), ¾ cup . . . .   1.0 d
  (La Choy Bi-Pack),* ¾ cup . . . .   2.0 d
  mix, prepared *(La Choy* Dinner Classics),
    ¾ cup . . . .   <1.0 d
Chicken entree, frozen:
breast, strips, mesquite *(Tyson),* 2.75 oz.   0
parmigiana *(Celentano),* 9 oz. . . . .   4.0 d
primavera *(Celentano),* 11.5 oz. . . . .   7.0 d

wings, all varieties *(Tyson)*, 3.5 oz. 0
wings, hot *(Weaver)*, 2.7 oz. 0
Chicken entree, refrigerated:
barbecue or roasted, all varieties *(Perdue Done It!)* 1 oz. 0
wings, hot and spicy *(Perdue Done It!)*, 1 oz. 0
Chicken fat* 0
Chicken frankfurter:
plain or with cheese, 4 oz. 0
Chicken giblets or gizzards:
all varieties* 0
Chicken gravy, canned:
(Heinz HomeStyle), 1/4 cup . . . . .4 d
with mushroom and onion *(Heinz* HomeStyle), 1/4 cup 0
Chicken liver* 0
Chicken liver pâté:
canned, 1 oz. . . . . <.1 d
Chicken luncheon meat:
all varieties, 8 oz. 0
Chicken salad spread:
(Libby's Spreadables), 1.9 oz. . . . . 1.0 d
Chicken teriyaki:
(La Choy Bi-Pack), 3/4 cup . . . . 1.0 d
Chickpea flour:
(Arrowhead Mills), 2 oz. . . . . 7.4 d
Chickpeas, dry:
uncooked:
  1 oz. . . . . 4.9 d
  1/2 cup . . . . 17.4 d
  (Arrowhead Mills), 2 oz. . . . . 7.0 d
boiled, 1/2 cup . . . . 2.9 d
Chickpeas, canned:
with liquid, 4 oz. . . . . 5.0 d
with liquid, 1/2 cup . . . . 5.3 d

Chickpeas, canned *(cont.)*

(Allens), ¹/₂ cup	4.0 d
(Eden), ¹/₂ cup	4.0 d
(Eden No Salt Added), ¹/₂ cup	4.0 d
(Green Giant/Joan of Arc), ¹/₂ cup	5.0 d
(Hain), 4 oz.	6.0 d
(Progresso), 4 oz.	6.0 d

Chicory, witloof, fresh:

untrimmed, 1 lb.	12.5 d
1 head, 5″ to 7″ long, approximately 2.1 oz. untrimmed	1.6 d
trimmed, ¹/₂ cup	1.4 d

Chicory greens, fresh:

untrimmed, 1 lb.	14.9 d
trimmed, 1 oz.	1.1 d
trimmed, chopped, ¹/₂ cup	3.6 d

Chicory root:

untrimmed, 1 lb.	7.3 c
1 medium, approximately 2.6 oz. untrimmed	1.2 c
trimmed, 1″ pieces, ¹/₂ cup	.9 c

Chili, canned or packaged:

with beans:

4 oz.	5.0 d
¹/₂ cup	5.6 d
(Gebhardt), 1 cup	6.0 d
(Just Rite), 4 oz.	1.0 d
(Old El Paso), 1 cup	6.0 d
hot *(Gebhardt)*, 1 cup	6.0 d
hot *(Just Rite)*, 4 oz.	1.0 d
without beans *(Gebhardt)*, 1 cup	1.0 d
without beans *(Just Rite)*, 4 oz.	<1.0 d
vegetarian, mild, 3 bean *(Health Valley* Fat Free), 5 oz.	9.0 d
vegetarian, mild or spicy, with black beans *(Health Valley* Fat Free), 5 oz.	12.2 d

Chili, frozen:
with beans, meatless *(Bodin's)*, 4 oz. . . . . 1.0 d
Chili, mix, prepared:
(Fantastic Cha-Cha Chili), 10 oz. . . . . 13.0 d
(Hunt's Manwich Chili Fixin's), 8 oz. . . . . 5.0 d
black bean *(Aunt Patsy's Super Black Bean)*,
    8 oz. . . . . 5.0 d
lentil *(Aunt Patsy's Pantry)*, 8 oz. . . . . 6.0 d
vegetarian *(Fantastic)*, 4 oz. . . . . 2.4 d
Chili beans, canned:
(Gebhardt), 4 oz. 5.0 d
(Green Giant/Joan of Arc 50% Less Salt),
    ½ cup . . . . 7.0 d
(Hunt's), 4 oz. . . . . 6.0 d
extra spicy *(Green Giant/Joan of Arc)*, ½ cup . . . 6.0 d
hot *(Campbell's)*, 4 oz. . . . . 5.0 d
spicy *(Green Giant/Joan of Arc)*, ½ cup . . . . . . 7.0 d
Chili pepper, see "Pepper, chili"
Chili powder:
1 oz. . . . . 9.7 d
1 tbsp. . . . . 2.6 d
1 tsp. . . . . .9 d
(Gebhardt), 1 tsp. <1.0 d
Chili sauce:
(Tabasco 7 Spice), 1 oz. . . . . .6 d
hot dog *(Gebhardt)*, 2 tbsp. . . . . <1.0 d
hot dog *(Just Rite)*, 2 oz. . . . . <1.0 d
red *(Las Palmas)*, ½ cup 0
spicy *(Tabasco 7 Spice)*, 1 oz. . . . . .6 d
Chili seasoning mix:
(Gebhardt Chili Quik), 1 tsp. . . . . <1.0 d
(Lawry's Seasoning Blends), 1 package . . . . 2.1 c
(Old El Paso), ⅕ package . . . . 1.0 d
(Tio Sancho), 1.23 oz. . . . . 4.2 c
Chinese perserving melon, see "Wax gourd"
Chitterlings, pork* 0

Chives, fresh:

1 oz. . . . . .9 d

chopped, ¼ cup . . . . .3 d

chopped, 1 tbsp. . . . . .1 d

Chocolate, see "Candy"

Chocolate, baking:

chips, semisweet or milk, maxi *(Guittard)*, 1 oz. . <1.0 d

chips, semisweet, mint, or mini *(Nestlé* Toll

   House Morsels), 1 oz. . . . . 4.0 d

squares, unsweetened, 1 oz. . . . . 4.7 d

premelted, unsweetened, 1-oz. packet . . . . .9 c

shreds *(Tone's),* 1 tsp. . . . . .1 d

Chocolate drink or milk:

regular or lowfat, 8 fl. oz. . . . . (0)

Chocolate flavor drink mix:

3 heaping tsp. . . . . 1.3 d

Chocolate syrup:

thin type, 1 tbsp. . . . . .3 d

Chocolate topping:

fudge type, 1 tbsp. .3 d

Chow mein, see "Beef chow mein," "Chicken

   entree," "Shrimp chow mein," and

   "Vegetable chow mein"

Chow mein noodles, see "Noodles, Chinese"

Chrysanthemum garland:

raw:

  untrimmed, 1 lb. 12.6 d

  1 stem, 8¾" long, approximately ½ oz.

    untrimmed . . . . .4 d

   trimmed, 1" pieces, ½ cup . . . . .4 d

boiled, drained, 1" pieces, ½ cup . . . . 1.2 d

Cilantro, see "Coriander"

Cinnamon, ground:

1 oz. . . . . 15.4 d

1 tsp. . . . . 1.2 d

Cisco* 0

Citrus grill marinade:
(Lawry's), 2 tbsp. . . . . .1 c
Citrus juice drink or punch:
bottled, 6 fl. oz. . . . . - (0)
frozen concentrate, undiluted, 6-fl.-oz. can . . . . . . .2 d
Clams* 0
Clam chowder, see "Soup"
Clam juice:
canned or bottled 0
Clover seeds, sprouted:
raw *(Shaw's)*, 2 oz. 3.0 d
Cloves, ground:
1 oz. . . . . 9.7 d
1 tbsp. . . . . 2.1 d
1 tsp. . . . . .7 d
Club soda:
plain or flavored 0
Cobbler:
apple, deep dish *(Awrey's)*, ⅛ pie . . . . 1.0 d
blueberry, deep dish *(Awrey's)*, ⅛ pie . . . . 2.0 d
Cobbler, frozen:
apple or peach *(Stilwell)*, ½ cup . . . . 3.0 d
apricot or blackberry *(Stilwell)*, ½ cup . . . . 5.0 d
cherry *(Stilwell)*, ½ cup . . . . 2.0 d
pecan or strawberry *(Stilwell)*, ½ cup . . . . 4.0 d
Cocktail sauce, seafood:
(Heinz), ¼ cup 0
Cocoa powder:
unsweetened, 1 tbsp. 1.6 d
Cocoa mix, 1 packet, except as noted:
1-oz. packet . . . . .3 d
all varieties *(Swiss Miss/Swiss Miss Lite)*,
  1 packet 0
chocolate, all varieties *(Carnation)*, 1 packet . . . . . . (0)
Coconut, fresh:
in shell, 1 lb. . . . . 21.2 d

Coconut *(cont.)*
shelled:

1 oz.	2.6 d
1 piece, 2″ × 2″ × ½″, approximately 1.6 oz.	4.1 d
shredded or grated, ½ cup not packed	3.6 d

Coconut, canned:

sweetened, flaked, 1 oz.	1.3 d
sweetened, flaked, ½ cup	1.7 d

Coconut, packaged:

sweetened, flaked, 1 oz.	1.2 d
sweetened, flaked, ½ cup	.9 d

dried:

sweetened, shredded, 1 oz.	1.3 d
sweetened, shredded, ½ cup	2.1 d
toasted, 1 oz.	.7 c

Coconut bar:

frozen *(Sunkist)*, 1 bar	1.4 c

Coconut cream, canned, sweetened:

1 oz.	.6 d
½ cup	3.3 d
1 tbsp.	.4 d

Coconut milk[1]:

1 oz.	.6 d
½ cup	2.6 d
1 tbsp.	.3 d

Coconut oil:

all varieties	0

Coconut water[2]:

1 oz.	.3 d
½ cup	1.3 d
1 tbsp.	.2 d

Cod* 0
Cod, canned and salted 0

[1] Liquid expressed from mixture of grated coconut and water.
[2] Liquid from coconuts.

Cod liver oil:

plain or flavored 0

Cod nuggets:

frozen *(Frionor Bunch O'Crunch)*, 8 nuggets,

    4 oz. . . . . <.1 d

Coffee:

regular or decaffeinated, brewed, 1 cup 0

freeze-dried or instant, prepared, 1 cup 0

Coffee, flavored (see also "Cappuccino"):

all varieties *(General Foods* International),

    6 fl. oz. . . . . (0)

all varieties *(Hills Bros.)*, 6 fl. oz. . . . . (0)

Coffee cake, see "Cake" and "Cake, snack"

Coffee creamer (whitener):

dairy or nondairy, 1 tbsp. 0

Coffee liqueur:

all varieties 0

Coffee substitute, cereal grain:

mix, whole grain, 1 tsp. . . . . .3 d

instant, prepared, all varieties *(Postum)*, 6 fl. oz. . . . (0)

Cognac:

plain or flavored 0

Cola, soda:

regular or diet, plain or flavored 0

Cold cuts, see specific listings

Collards, fresh:

raw:

    untrimmed, 1 lb. . . . . 9.6 d

    trimmed, 1 oz. . . . . 1.0 d

    trimmed, chopped, ½ cup . . . . .7 d

boiled, drained, chopped, ½ cup . . . . 1.3 d

Collards, frozen:

unheated, 3.3 oz., ⅓ of 10-oz. package . . . . . . 1.9 d

chopped, boiled, drained, ½ cup . . . . .9 c

Cookies:

almond biscuit *(Almondina)*, 1 piece . . . . .4 d

apple filled *(Archway)*, 1 piece 0

apple n' raisin *(Archway)*, 1 piece . . . . 1.0 d

apple-raisin filled *(Health Valley Fruit Centers)*,
  1 piece . . . . 3.5 d

apple or apricot filled *(Health Valley Fruit
  Centers)*, 1 piece . . . . 2.0 d

apricot or blueberry filled *(Archway)*, 1 piece . . . . 1.0 d

brownie, see "Brownies"

butter pecan *(Dare)*, 1 piece . . . . .1 d

caramel, golden *(Dare)*, 1 piece . . . . .1 d

carob chip *(Health Valley Healthy Chip)*,
  1.17 oz. or 3 pieces . . . . 3.0 d

carrot cake *(Archway)*, 1 piece 0

(Carr's Hob Nobs), 1 piece . . . . .7 d

cherry filled *(Archway)*, 1 piece . . . . 1.0 d

chocolate fudge *(Dare)*, 1 piece . . . . .3 d

chocolate, milk, fudge *(Dare)*, 1 piece . . . . .2 d

chocolate chip or chunk:

  (Archway Mini)*, 12 pieces 0

  (Archway Super Pak)*, 1 piece . . . . 1.0 d

  (Dare), 1 piece .2 d

  (Dare Breaktime)*, 1 piece . . . . .1 d

  (Hostess), 5 pieces . . . . 2.0 d

  (Pepperidge Farm Family Request)*, 2 pieces . 1.0 d

  bar *(Tastykake)*, 1 piece . . . . 1.0 d

  chocolate walnut *(Pepperidge Farm* Beacon
    Hill)*, 1 piece . . . . 1.0 d

  chunk *(Pepperidge Farm* Nantucket)*, 1 piece . 1.0 d

  chunk, macadamia *(Tastykake)*, 1 piece . . . . . . 2.0 d

  chunk, pecan *(Pepperidge Farm*
    Chesapeake)*, 1 piece . . . . 1.0 d

  drop *(Archway)*, 1 piece . . . . .5 d

  milk *(Dare* Jersey Milk Chip)*, 1 piece . . . . .1 d

milk, macadamia *(Pepperidge Farm
    Sausalito),* 1 piece 0
toffee *(Archway),* 1 piece . . . . 1.0 d
chocolate sandwich *(Famous Amos),* 3 pieces . . . 1.0 d
chocolate snap *(Archway),* 6 pieces 0
chocolate, sugar *(Pepperidge Farm* Family
    Request), 2 pieces 0
cocoa, Dutch *(Archway),* 1 piece 0
coconut:
  (Dare Breaktime), 1 piece . . . . .1 d
  creme *(Dare),* 1 piece . . . . .2 d
  macaroon *(Archway),* 1 piece . . . . 3.0 d
(Dare Harvest from the Rain Forest), 1 piece . . . . . .2 d
date filled *(Health Valley Fruit Centers),* 1 piece . 3.5 d
fig bar, 1 piece, approximately .6 oz. . . . . .7 d
fortune *(La Choy),* 1 piece . . . . <1.0 d
French creme *(Dare),* 1 piece . . . . .2 d
fruit (see also specific fruit cookie listings):
  all varieties *(Health Valley* Fat Free Jumbo
      Fruit Cookies), 1 piece . . . . 2.0 d
  chunks, all varieties *(Health Valley* Fat Free),
      3 pieces . . . . 3.0 d
  tropical, filled *(Health Valley Fruit Centers),*
      1 piece . . . . 2.0 d
fruit cake *(Archway),* 3 pieces . . . . 2.0 d
fruit filled, all varieties *(Health Valley Mini Fruit
    Centers* Fat Free), 3 pieces . . . . 3.0 d
fruit and honey bar *(Archway),* 1 piece . . . . 1.0 d
fudge bar *(Tastykake),* 1 piece . . . . 1.0 d
fudge nut bar *(Archway),* 1 piece . . . . 1.0 d
gingersnaps *(Archway),* 6 pieces . . . . 1.0 d
graham cracker *(Carr's* Home Wheat), 1 piece . . . . .4 d
graham cracker, dark or milk chocolate *(Carr's*
    Home Wheat), 1 piece . . . . .3 d
ladyfingers, 4 pieces 0

Cookies (cont.)

lemon, frosty (Archway), 1 piece	0
lemon creme (Dare), 1 piece	.2 d
lemon snaps (Archway), 6 pieces	1.0 d
maple-leaf creme (Dare), 1 piece	.3 d
maple-walnut fudge (Dare), 1 piece	.2 d
marshmallow cake, all flavors (Dare Belmont Mallow), 1 piece	.1 d
mint (Dare Midnight Mint), 1 piece	.1 d
molasses (Archway Old Fashioned), 1 piece	0
molasses, plain or iced (Archway), 1 piece	1.0 d
New Orleans cake (Archway), 1 piece	1.0 d
nougat, nutty (Archway), 3 pieces	0
oat-bran raisin (Awrey's), 1 piece	1.0 d

oatmeal:

(Archway), 1 piece	1.0 d
(Archway Mini), 12 pieces	1.0 d
(Dare Breaktime), 1 piece	.2 d
(Pepperidge Farm Family Request), 2 pieces	1.0 d
chocolate (Pepperidge Farm Dakota), 1 piece	1.0 d
date filled or iced (Archway), 1 piece	1.0 d
golden (Archway Ruth's),	1.0 d

oatmeal raisin:

(Archway), 1 piece	1.0 d
(Dare), 1 piece	.5 d
(Pepperidge Farm Santa Fe), 1 piece	1.0 d
bar (Tastykake), 1 piece	1.0 d
bran (Archway), 1 piece	1.0 d
orange, frosty (Archway), 1 piece	0

peanut butter:

(Archway), 1 piece	1.0 d
(Dare Peanut Butter Delites), 1 piece	.2 d
(Pepperidge Farm Family Request), 2 pieces	1.0 d
N' chips (Archway), 1 piece	1.0 d
chip (Dare), 1 piece	.1 d

chocolate chip *(Pepperidge Farm* Cheyenne),
  1 piece . . . . 1.0 d
nougat *(Archway),* 3 pieces . . . . 1.0 d
pecan:
  crunch *(Archway),* 1 piece . . . . 1.0 d
  ice box *(Archway),* 1 piece 0
  nougat, malted *(Archway),* 3 pieces . . . . 2.0 d
pineapple filled *(Archway),* 1 piece . . . . 1.0 d
raisin oatmeal *(Archway),* 1 piece . . . . 1.0 d
raisin oatmeal *(Dare Sun Maid* Raisin Oatmeal),
  1 piece . . . . .3 d
raspberry filled *(Archway),* 1 piece . . . . 1.0 d
raspberry filled *(Health Valley Fruit Centers),*
  1 piece . . . . 2.0 d
rocky road *(Archway),* 1 piece . . . . 1.0 d
shortbread, butter *(Dare),* 1 piece . . . . .2 d
strawberry filled *(Archway),* 1 piece . . . . 1.0 d
sugar:
  (Archway), 1 piece 0
  drop, soft *(Archway),* 1 piece 0
  wafer, vanilla *(Tastykake),* 1 piece 0
tea biscuit *(Dare* Social Tea), 1 piece . . . . .3 d
wedding cake *(Archway),* 3 pieces . . . . .0 d
wheat *(Carr's Wheatolo),* 1 piece . . . . .4 d
wheatmeal, large *(Carr's),* 1 piece . . . . .9 d
wheatmeal, small *(Carr's),* 1 piece . . . . .5 d
windmill *(Archway* Old Fashioned), 1 piece 0
Coquito nut:
shelled *(Frieda's),* 1 oz. . . . . 3.4 d
Coriander, fresh:
untrimmed, 1 lb. . . . . 8.9 d
9 plants, approximately .8 oz. . . . . .5 d
½ cup . . . . .2 d
Coriander, dried:
1 oz. . . . . 2.9 d
1 tsp. . . . . .1 d

Coriander seeds:

dried, 1 tsp. . . . . .5 c

Corn, fresh:

raw:

   on the cob, with husks, untrimmed, 1 lb. . . . . . 4.4 d

   kernels, 4 oz. 3.1 d

   kernels, ½ cup . . . . 2.1 d

boiled, drained, 1 ear, approximately 2.7 oz. . . . . 2.2 d

boiled, drained, kernels, ½ cup . . . . 2.3 d

Corn, canned:

kernels:

   (Comstock), ½ cup . . . . 2.0 d

   (Green Giant Delicorn/Niblets), ½ cup . . . . . . 2.0 d

   (Green Giant Sweet Select), ½ cup . . . . 3.0 d

   with liquid, 4 oz. . . . . .8 d

   with liquid, ½ cup . . . . .9 d

   drained, ½ cup . . . . 1.6 d

   vacuum pack, 4 oz. . . . . 6.5 d

   vacuum pack, ½ cup . . . . 6.0 d

   golden or white, sweet *(Green Giant),* ½ cup . 2.0 d

   with peppers *(Green Giant Mexicorn),* ½ cup . 3.0 d

cream style:

   4 oz. . . . . 1.4 d

   ½ cup . . . . 1.5 d

   (Green Giant), ½ cup . . . . 2.0 d

Corn, frozen:

on the cob:

   1 ear, approximately 4 oz. . . . . 1.5 d

   (Green Giant Nibblers), 2 ears . . . . 2.0 d

   (Green Giant Nibblers One Serving),

     2 half ears . . . . 2.0 d

   (Green Giant Niblet Ears/Sweet Select), 1 ear . 2.0 d

   (Green Giant Sweet Select Half Ears),* 2 ears . 2.0 d

kernels:

   unheated, 3.3 oz. . . . . 2.3 d

½ cup	2.0 d
(Green Giant Harvest Fresh Niblets), ½ cup ...	2.0 d
(Green Giant Nibblets/Sweet Select), ½ cup ...	2.0 d
white shoepeg *(Green Giant Harvest Fresh/*	
Select), ½ cup	2.0 d
cream-style *(Green Giant)*, ½ cup	2.5 d
in butter sauce:	
(Green Giant Niblets), ½ cup	2.0 d
(Green Giant Niblets One Serving), 4.5 oz.	3.0 d
white shoepeg *(Green Giant)*, ½ cup	2.0 d

Corn, packaged:

with green beans, carrots, and pasta *(Green*	
Giant Pantry Express), ½ cup	3.0 d

Corn, whole grain:

blue *(Arrowhead Mills)*, 2 oz.	5.6 d
yellow *(Arrowhead Mills)*, 2 oz.	6.8 d

Corn bran, crude:

1 oz.	24.4 d
½ cup	32.7 d
1 tbsp.	4.1 d

Corn chips, puffs, and similar snacks, 1 oz.:

all varieties *(Fritos)*	1.1 d
all varieties *(Santitas)*	1.5 d
cheese:	
(Cheddar Valley)	1.0 d
all varieties *(Chee·tos)*	1.0 d
(Health Valley Cheese Puffs)	2.2 d
hot *(Flamin' Hot)*	1.0 d
tortilla, see "Tortilla chips"	

Corn flake crumbs:

(Kellogg's), 1 oz.	1.0 d

Corn flour:

whole grain, 2 oz.	7.6 d
whole grain, ½ cup	7.8 d
masa, 2 oz.	5.4 d
masa, ½ cup	5.5 d

Corn grits (see also "Hominy"), dry:

instant *(Quaker Original)*, 1 oz. . . . .   1.5 d

white or yellow *(Arrowhead Mills)*, 2 oz. . . . .   1.5 d

Corn oil:

all varieties   0

Corn syrup:

all varieties, 1 cup   0

Corn bread, see "Bread, corn"

Cornish game hen*   0

Cornish game hen, roasted, all varieties

   (Perdue Done It!)   0

Cornmeal (see also "Corn flour" and "Polenta

   mix"):

whole grain, 2 oz. . . . .   4.1 d

whole grain, ½ cup . . . .   4.5 d

degermed, 2 oz. . . . .   4.2 d

degermed, ½ cup . . . .   5.1 d

blue *(Arrowhead Mills)*, 2 oz. . . . .   5.6 d

white or yellow *(Albers)*, 1 oz. . . . .   1.5 d

yellow or hi-lysine *(Arrowhead Mills)*, 2 oz. . . . . .   6.8 d

Cornmeal mix:

white *(Aunt Jemima)*, 1 oz. . . . .   3.0 d

Cornstarch:

1 oz. . . . .   .3 d

1 tbsp. . . . .   .1 d

Cottonseed kernels, roasted:

1 oz. . . . .   1.6 d

½ cup . . . .   4.1 d

1 tbsp. . . . .   .6 d

Cottonseed meal:

partially defatted, 1 oz. . . . .   .7 c

Cottonseed oil:

all varieties   0

Cough drops, see "Candy"

Couscous:

uncooked, 1 oz.	1.4 d
uncooked, ½ cup	4.6 d
cooked, ½ cup	1.3 d

Couscous mix*:

(Fantastic Foods), ½ cup	2.6 d
pilaf, savory (Quick Pilaf), ½ cup	3.0 d
whole wheat (Fantastic Foods), ½ cup	3.0 d

Cowpeas, immature seeds, fresh:

raw, untrimmed, 1 lb.	11.6 d
raw, trimmed, ½ cup	3.6 d
boiled, drained, ½ cup	4.1 d
leafy tips, raw, chopped, ½ cup	.2 c
leafy tips, boiled, drained, 4 oz.	3.0 c
pods, with seeds, raw or boiled and drained, ½ cup	.8 c

Cowpeas, canned:

(Allens/East Texas Fair), ½ cup	4.0 d
with jalapeños (Home-Folks), ½ cup	4.0 d

Cowpeas, frozen:

unheated, 3.3 oz.	4.7 d
boiled, drained, ½ cup	4.3 d

Cowpeas, mature, dry:

uncooked, 1 oz.	3.0 d
uncooked, ½ cup	8.9 d
boiled, ½ cup	5.6 d

Cowpeas, mature, canned:

with liquid, 4 oz.	3.8 d
with liquid, ½ cup	4.0 d
(Allens/East Texas Fair), ½ cup	2.0 d
(Green Giant/Joan of Arc), ½ cup	4.0 d
with bacon (Allens/Sunshine), ½ cup	2.0 d
with pork, 4 oz. or ½ cup	4.0 d

Cowpeas, catjang, see "Catjang"

Crab* 0

"Crab," imitation:

made from surimi 0

(*Louis Kemp* Crab DeLights), 2 oz. 0

Crabapple:

fresh, unpeeled, 4 oz. . . . . .7 d

Cracker crumbs, see "Matzo crumbs"

Crackers:

butter flavor (*Carr's* Butterpuff), 1 piece . . . . .3 d

butter thins (*Pepperidge Farm*), 4 pieces 0

cheddar (*Carr's*), 1 piece . . . . .1 d

cheese, three (*Pepperidge Farm* Snack Sticks),

  8 pieces . . . . 1.0 d

cheese sandwich:

crispbread (see also specific cracker listings):

  (*Wasa* Breakfast), 1 piece . . . . .7 d

  (*Wasa* Fiber Plus), 1 piece . . . . 2.8 d

  cinnamon sugar wheat (*Pepperidge Farm*),

    ½ oz. . . . . 1.0 d

  dark, regular or with caraway (*Finn Crisp*),

    2 pieces . . . . 1.6 d

  high fiber (*Ryvita* Crisp Bread), 1 piece . . . . . . 2.0 d

  high fiber (*Ryvita* Snackbread), 1 piece . . . . . . 1.0 d

croissant (*Carr's*), 1 piece . . . . .1 d

(*Dare Breton/Cabaret/Vivant*), 1 piece . . . . .1 d

flatbread:

  (*J.J. Flats* Flavorall), 1 piece . . . . 1.0 d

  all varieties, except plain, onion, and poppy

    (*J.J. Flats*), 1 piece . . . . 1.0 d

  plain, onion, and poppy (*J.J. Flats*), 1 piece . . . <1.0 d

matzo:

  plain, 1 oz. . . . . .9 d

  regular, unsalted, and tea thin (*Manischewitz*

    Daily), 1 board . . . . .1 d

  egg and onion, 1 oz. . . . . 1.4 d

  thin, regular or dietetic (*Manischewitz*),

    1 board . . . . .1 d

whole wheat, 1 oz. . . . . 3.4 d
whole wheat with bran *(Manischewitz)*,
  1 board . . . . .6 d
melba toast:
  plain, 1 oz. . . . . 1.8 d
  rye or pumpernickel, 1 oz. . . . . 2.3 d
  wheat, 1 oz. . . . . 2.1 d
oat bran *(Oat Bran Krisp)*, 1/2 oz. . . . . 3.2 d
pizza flavor *(Pepperidge Farm Goldfish)*, 1/2 oz. . 1.0 d
poppy and sesame seed *(Carr's)*, 1 piece . . . . . . .1 d
pretzel or pumpernickel *(Pepperidge Farm*
  Snack Sticks), 8 pieces . . . . 1.0 d
rye:
  (Rykrisp), 1/2 oz. . . . . 3.6 d
  crispbread, 2 pieces, approximately .7 oz. . . . . 3.2 d
  dark or light *(Ryvita Crisp Bread)*, 1 piece . . . . 1.3 d
  light *(Wasa Crispbread)*, 1 piece . . . . 1.2 d
  seasoned or sesame *(Rykrisp)*, 1/2 oz. . . . . 3.0 d
  sesame, toasted *(Ryvita Crisp Bread)*, 1 piece . 1.4 d
saltines, 1 oz., approximately 9 pieces . . . . .8 d
sesame:
  (Dare Breton), 1 piece . . . . .1 d
  (Pepperidge Farm), 4 pieces . . . . 2.0 d
  (Pepperidge Farm Snack Sticks), 8 pieces . . . . 1.0 d
soda or water:
  1 oz. . . . . .8 d
  (Pepperidge Farm English Water Biscuit),
    4 pieces 0
  bite-size or oblong *(Carr's Table Water)*,
    1 piece . . . . .1 d
  king-size *(Carr's Table Water)*, 1 piece . . . . .3 d
  with cracked pepper or sesame seeds *(Carr's*
    Table Water), 1 piece . . . . .1 d
soup and oyster, 1/2 oz., approximately 14 small
  pieces . . . . .4 d

Crackers *(cont.)*
soup and oyster *(Carr's* Scalloped Round),
  1 piece . . . . .1 d
wheat:
  (Ryvita Original Snackbread), 1 piece . . . . .2 d
  cracked *(Pepperidge Farm),* 3 pieces . . . . 1.0 d
  grain *(Carr's),* 1 piece . . . . .3 d
  hearty or toasted with onion *(Pepperidge
    Farm),* 4 pieces . . . . 1.0 d
wheat, whole *(Carr's* Star), 1 piece . . . . .2 d
wheat, whole *(Carr's* Wheatmeal), 1 piece . . . . . . .5 d
Cranberry beans, dry:
boiled, 1/2 cup . . . . 3.0 d
Cranberry beans, canned:
with liquid, 1/2 cup . . . . 1.2 c
Cranberry fruit concentrate:
(Hain), 2 tbsp. . . . . <1.0 d
Cranberry juice cocktail:
bottled, 6 fl.-oz. . . . . .2 d
frozen concentrate, undiluted, 6-fl.-oz. can . . . . . . .4 d
low-calorie, bottled, 6 fl. oz. 0
Cranberry sauce, canned:
whole or jellied, 4 oz. . . . . 1.1 d
whole or jellied, 1/2 cup . . . . 1.4 d
Cranberry-apple juice drink:
bottled, 6 fl. oz. . . . . .2 d
Cranberry-apricot juice drink:
bottled, 6 fl. oz. . . . . .2 d
Cranberry-grape juice drink:
bottled, 6 fl. oz. . . . . .2 d
Cranberry-orange relish:
canned, 1/2 cup . . . . .8 c
Cranberries, fresh, raw:
whole, 4 oz. . . . . 4.8 d
whole, 1/2 cup . . . . 2.0 d
chopped, 1/2 cup . . . . 2.3 d

Crayfish* 0
Cream:
dairy or nondairy, all varieties 0
Cream, sour:
dairy or nondairy, regular or light 0
light, with chives *(Land O'Lakes)*, 2 tbsp. . . . . (0)
Cream peas, see "Peas, cream"
Cream puff, Bavarian:
frozen *(Rich's)*, 1 piece 0
Cream of tartar:
(Tone's), 1 tbsp. 0
Cream topping:
dairy or nondairy 0
Crème liqueurs:
all varieties (de cassis, framboise, de menthe) 0
Cress, garden, fresh:
raw, untrimmed, 1 lb. . . . . 3.5 d
raw, ½ cup . . . . .3 d
boiled, drained, ½ cup . . . . .5 d
Cress, water, see "Watercress"
Croaker* 0
Croissant:
butter, 1 medium, approximately 2 oz. . . . . 1.6 d
butter *(Awrey's)*, 3 oz. piece . . . . 1.0 d
apple, 1 medium, approximately 2 oz. . . . . 1.4 d
cheese, 1 medium, approximately 2 oz. . . . . 2.2 d
margarine *(Awrey's)*, 2.5-oz. piece . . . . 1.0 d
wheat *(Awrey's)*, 1 piece . . . . 1.0 d
Crookneck squash, fresh:
raw, untrimmed, 1 lb. 8.2 d
raw, sliced, ½ cup . . . . 1.2 d
boiled, drained, sliced, ½ cup . . . . 1.3 d
Crookneck squash, canned:
drained, 4 oz. . . . . 1.1 d
drained, cut, ½ cup . . . . 1.1 d

Crookneck squash, frozen:

unheated, 3.3 oz.	1.1 d
unheated, ½ cup	.8 d
frozen, boiled, sliced, ½ cup	1.2 d

Croutons:

plain, ½ oz.	.7 d
plain, ½ cup	.8 d
Caesar salad *(Brownberry)*, ½ oz.	<1.0 d
cheddar or cheese and garlic *(Brownberry)*, ½ oz.	<1.0 d
cheese and garlic or Italian *(Arnold* Crispy), ½ oz.	<1.0 d
fine herb *(Arnold* Crispy), ½ oz.	1.0 d
onion and garlic or wheat *(Brownberry)*, ½ oz.	1.0 d
ranch *(Pepperidge Farm)*, ½ oz.	1.0 d
seasoned:	
½ oz.	.7 d
½ cup	1.0 d
(Arnold), ½ oz.	<1.0 d
seasoned or toasted *(Brownberry)*, ½ oz.	<1.0 d

Crowder peas, fresh, see "Cowpeas"

Crowder peas, canned:

(Allens/East Texas Fair), ½ cup	4.0 d

Cucumber, unpeeled:

untrimmed, 1 lb.	3.5 d
1 medium, 8¼″ long, approximately 11 oz.	2.4 d
sliced, ½ cup	.4 d

Cumin seeds:

1 oz.	3.0 d
1 tsp.	.2 d

Cupcake, see "Cake, snack"

Currants, trimmed:

black, European, 4 oz.	6.2 d
black, European, ½ cup	3.0 d
red and white, 4 oz.	4.9 d
red and white, ½ cup	2.4 d

zante, dried, 2 oz. . . . . 3.8 d
zante, dried, ½ cup . . . . 4.9 d
Curry powder:
1 oz. . . . . 9.4 d
1 tbsp. . . . . 2.2 d
1 tsp. . . . . .7 d
Curry sauce mix:
1.25-oz. packet . . . . .5 c
Cusk* 0
Custard, egg:
1 cup 0
Custard apple:
trimmed, 1 oz. . . . . 1.0 c
Cuttlefish* 0

D

Food and Measure	Fiber Grams

Daikon, see "Radish, Oriental"
Daiquiri cocktail mixer:
bottled, all varieties *(Holland House),* 3 fl. oz. . . . . . (0)
Dandelion greens, fresh:
raw, 1 lb. . . . . 15.9 d
raw, chopped, ½ cup . . . . 1.0 d
boiled, drained, chopped, ½ cup . . . . 1.5 d
Danish pastry:
all varieties *(Awrey's),* 1 piece . . . . 1.0 d
cinnamon, 1 piece, 4½" diameter,
   approximately 2.3 oz. . . . . .8 d
fruit[1], 1 piece, 4¼" diameter, approximately
   2.5 oz. . . . . 1.3 d
nut[2], 1 piece, 4¼" diameter, approximately
   2.3 oz. . . . . 1.5 d
Dasheen, see "Taro"
Date-nut bread, see "Bread, date nut"
Date-nut pastry, see "Cake, snack"
Dates, pitted:
(Bordo), 2 oz. . . . . 1.5 c
diced *(Bordo),* 2 oz. . . . . 1.2 c

---

[1] Includes apple, cinnamon raisin, lemon, raspberry, and strawberry.
[2] Includes almond, raisin nut, and cinnamon nut.

domestic, natural and dry:

2 oz.	4.2 d
10 dates, approximately 2.9 oz.	6.2 d
chopped, ½ cup	6.7 d

Dill seasoning:
(McCormick/Shilling Parsley Patch It's a Dilly),

½ tsp.	(0)

Dill seeds, dried:

1 oz.	6.0 d
1 tsp.	.4 d

Dill seeds, sprouted:

raw *(Shaw's)*, 2 oz.	3.0 d

Dill weed:

dried *(Tone's)*, 1 tsp.	.1 d

Dishcloth gourd:

raw, 1 gourd, 13¼" long, approximately 8.6 oz. untrimmed	1.7 c
boiled, drained, 1" slices, ½ cup	.4 d

Dock:

raw, untrimmed, 1 lb.	9.2 d
raw, chopped, ½ cup	1.9 d
boiled, drained, 4 oz.	.8 c

Dolphinfish* 0

Donuts:
plain:

(Awrey's)	1.0 d
(Hostess Breakfast Bake Shop Pantry)	.9 d
(Tastykake Assorted)	1.0 d
cake type, 1 medium, 2" diameter, approximately 1.7 oz.	.8 d

chocolate, sugared or glazed, 1 medium 3"

diameter, approximately 1.5 oz.	.9 d

chocolate frosted, 1 large, 3½" diameter,

approximately 2 oz.	1.1 d

cinnamon:

(Hostess Breakfast Bake Shop Donette Gems)	.3 d

Donuts, cinnamon *(cont.)*
  (Hostess Breakfast Bake Shop Pantry) . . . . .9 d
  (Tastykake Assorted) . . . . 1.0 d
  (Tastykake Mini) 0
  apple filled *(Hostess Breakfast Bake Shop*
    Donette Gems) .3 d
crumb *(Hostess Breakfast Bake Shop)* . . . . .9 d
crumb *(Hostess Breakfast Bake Shop Donette*
  Gems) . . . . .4 d
crunch *(Awrey's)* . . . . 2.0 d
frosted:
  (Hostess Breakfast Bake Shop) . . . . 1.1 d
  (Hostess Breakfast Bake Shop Donette Gems) . . .4 d
  (Hostess Breakfast Bake Shop O's) . . . . 1.7 d
  rich *(Tastykake)* . . . . 3.0 d
  rich *(Tastykake* Mini) . . . . 1.0 d
  strawberry filled *(Hostess Breakfast Bake*
    Shop Donette Gems) . . . . .5 d
glazed:
  (Hostess Breakfast Bake Shop Old
    Fashioned) . . . . 1.4 d
  whirl *(Hostess Breakfast Bake Shop)* . . . . .9 d
  yeast type, 1 medium, 3¾" diameter,
    approximately 2.1 oz. . . . . 1.3 d
honey wheat:
  (Hostess Breakfast Bake Shop) . . . . 1.2 d
  (Tastykake) . . . . 1.0 d
  (Tastykake Mini) 0
(Hostess Breakfast Bake Shop O's) . . . . 1.0 d
(Hostess Breakfast Bake Shop Old Fashioned) . . . . .9 d
orange glazed *(Tastykake)* . . . . 1.0 d
powdered sugar:
  (Awrey's) . . . . 2.0 d
  (Hostess Breakfast Bake Shop Assorted) . . . . . . .8 d
  (Hostess Breakfast Bake Shop Donette Gems) . . .2 d
  (Tastykake Assorted) . . . . 1.0 d

(Tastykake Mini)   0
strawberry filled *(Hostess Breakfast Bake
    Shop Donette Gems)* . . . . .3 d
Drum*
Duck*   0
Duck sauce, see "Sweet and sour sauce"
Dunkin' Donuts:
apple filled, cinnamon sugar, 1 piece . . . .   1.0 d
Bavarian cream filled, chocolate frosting,
    1 piece . . . .   2.0 d
blueberry filled, 1 piece . . . .   2.0 d
buttermilk ring, glazed, 1 piece . . . .   1.0 d
cake ring, plain, 1 piece . . . .   1.0 d
chocolate ring, glazed, 1 piece . . . .   1.9 d
coffee roll, glazed, 1 piece . . . .   2.0 d
cookie, chocolate chunk or oatmeal pecan
    raisin, 1 piece . . . .   1.0 d
cookie, chocolate chunk, with nuts, 1 piece . . . .   2.0 d
croissant, plain, 1 piece . . . .   2.0 d
croissant, almond or chocolate, 1 piece . . . .   3.0 d
French cruller, glazed, 1 piece   0
jelly or lemon filled, 1 piece . . . .   1.0 d
muffin:
    apple n' spice, 1 piece . . . .   2.0 d
    banana nut, 1 piece . . . .   3.0 d
    blueberry or cranberry nut, 1 piece . . . .   2.0 d
    bran, with raisins, 1 piece . . . .   4.0 d
    corn, 1 piece . . . .   1.0 d
    cranberry nut, 1 piece . . . .   2.0 d
    oat bran, 1 piece . . . .   3.0 d
whole wheat ring, glazed, 1 piece . . . .   2.0 d
yeast ring, chocolate frosted or glazed, 1 piece .   1.0 d
Dutch brand loaf:
(Kahn's), 1 slice . . . . (0)

E

Food and Measure	Fiber Grams

Eel* 0
Egg* 0
Egg, substitute or imitation:
frozen or refrigerated:
  (*Healthy Choice*), ¼ cup 0
  (*Morningstar Farms Better'n Eggs/*
    Scramblers), ¼ cup 0
  (*Second Nature*), 2 oz.................. 0
  plain or with "cheez" (*Fleischmann's Egg*
    Beaters), ¼ cup 0
mix, prepared (*Tofu Scrambler*), ½ cup ...... 2.3 d
Egg foo young mix, prepared:
(*La Choy* Dinner Classics), 2 patties and 3-oz.
  sauce .... 1.0 d
Eggnog:
(*Borden*), ½ cup 0
Eggnog flavor drink mix:
2 heaping tsp. .... .9 d
Eggplant, fresh:
raw:
  untrimmed, 1 lb. .... 9.2 d
  1 medium, peeled, approximately 1.2 lbs.
    untrimmed .... 11.5 d
  trimmed, 1" pieces, ½ cup .... 1.0 d
boiled, drained, 1" cubes, ½ cup .... 1.2 d

Eggplant appetizer:

baby, stuffed *(Krinos)*, 1.1 oz. . . . .   1.0 d

El Pollo Loco, 1 serving:

meals[1], steak or chicken fajita . . . .   17.0 d

chicken, all parts   0

burritos and tacos:

  chicken or steak burrito . . . .   4.0 d

  chicken or steak taco . . . .   2.0 d

  vegetarian burrito . . . .   7.0 d

salads and side dishes:

  beans . . . .   8.0 d

  chicken salad . . . .   4.0 d

  coleslaw . . . .   1.0 d

  corn . . . .   1.0 d

  corn or flour tortilla . . . .   <1.0 d

  guacamole, 1 oz.   0

  potato salad . . . .   1.0 d

  salsa, 2 oz. . . . .   1.0 d

  side salad . . . .   4.0 d

salad dressing, all varieties, 1 oz.   0

dessert:

  cheesecake   0

  churros   0

  Orange or Piña Colada Bang   0

Elderberries:

4 oz. . . . .   8.0 d

½ cup . . . .   5.1 d

Enchilada dinner mix:

(Tio Sancho Dinner Kit):

  sauce mix, 3 oz. . . . .   1.8 c

  1 shell . . . .   .6 c

Enchilada sauce:

(Gebhardt), 3 tbsp. . . . .   <1.0 d

mild *(Rosarita),* 2.5 oz. . . . .   <1.0 d

---

[1] Includes guacamole, cheese, and sour cream.

Enchilada sauce *(cont.)*
green *(Old El Paso)*, 2 tbsp. 0
hot *(Las Palmas)*, 1/2 cup 0
hot *(Old El Paso)*, 1/4 cup . . . . (0)
hot or mild *(Ortega)*, 1 oz. . . . . (0)
mild *(Old El Paso)*, 1/4 cup . . . . (0)
Enchilada seasoning mix:
(Lawry's Seasoning Blends), 1 package . . . . 1.4 c
(Old El Paso), 1/18 package 0
Endive, fresh, raw:
untrimmed, 1 lb. . . . . 12.1 d
1 head, approximately 1.3 lbs., untrimmed . . . . . 15.9 d
chopped, 1/2 cup . . . . .8 d
Endive, Belgian, see "Chicory, witloof"
Escarole, see "Endive"
Étouffée dinner mix:
(Luzianne), 1/4 package . . . . <1.0 d

F

Food and Measure	Fiber Grams

Fajita sauce:
(*Lawry's* Skillet Sauce), 1 oz. . . . . .1 c
Fajita seasoning mix:
(*Lawry's* Seasoning Blends), 1 package . . . . .5 c
Falafel mix:
(*Fantastic Falafel*), 3 oz. . . . . 7.0 d
Farina (see also "Cereal, cooking"), whole
  grain:
uncooked:
  2 oz. . . . . 1.5 d
  ½ cup . . . . 2.4 d
  1 tbsp. . . . . .5 d
cooked, ½ cup . . . . 1.6 d
cooked, 1 cup . . . . 3.3 d
Fat:
all varieties 0
Fava beans, see "Broad beans"
Fennel seeds:
1 oz. . . . . 4.4 c
1 tsp. . . . . .3 c
Fenugreek seeds:
1 oz. . . . . 2.9 c
1 tsp. . . . . .4 c
Fettuccine, see "Pasta"

Fettuccine Alfredo mix, prepared *(Hain Pasta & Sauce)*, ½ cup . . . . 1.5 d

Fettuccine primavera, frozen:

(Green Giant), 1 package . . . . 6.0 d

(Green Giant Garden Gourmet Right for Lunch), 9.5 oz. . . . . 6.0 d

Fiber supplement:

(FiberSonic), 1.35-oz. pouch . . . . 11.0 d

Field cress, see "Cress, garden"

Figs, fresh:

4 oz. . . . . 3.8 d

1 large, approximately 2.3 oz. . . . . 2.1 d

1 medium, approximately 1.8 oz. . . . . 1.7 d

Figs, canned:

in water or heavy syrup, 4 oz. . . . . 2.5 d

in water, 3 figs and 1¾ tbsp. liquid . . . . 1.8 d

in water, ½ cup . . . . 2.7 d

in light syrup:

    4 oz. . . . . 2.1 d

    3 figs and 1¾ tbsp. liquid . . . . 1.5 d

    ½ cup . . . . 2.3 d

in heavy syrup, 3 figs and 1¾ tbsp. liquid . . . . . 1.9 d

in heavy syrup, ½ cup . . . . 2.8 d

Figs, dried:

uncooked:

    2 oz. . . . . 5.2 d

    10 figs, approximately 6.6 oz. . . . . 17.4 d

    ½ cup . . . . 9.3 d

    Calamata string *(Agora)*, ½ cup . . . . 17.0 d

stewed, ½ cup . . . . 6.2 d

Filberts:

dried, unblanched:

    in shell, 1 lb. . . . . 12.7 d

    shelled, 1 oz. . . . . 1.7 d

    whole, ½ cup . . . . 4.1 d

chopped, 1/2 cup	7.5 d
ground, 1/2 cup	2.3 d
dry-roasted, 1 oz.	1.1 d
oil-roasted, 1 oz.	1.8 d
Finnan haddie*	0
Fish (see also specific listings)*	0
Fish batter seasoning mix:	
Cajun *(Tone's),* 1 tsp.	.1 d
Fish oil:	
all varieties, plain or flavored	0
Fish seasoning mix, see "Seafood seasoning mix"	
Fish sticks:	
breaded, frozen *(Frionor Bunch O'Crunch),* 4 pieces	<.1 d
Five spice, see "Oriental 5-spice"	
Flan:	
1 cup	0
Flatfish*	0
Flavor enhancer:	
(Ac'cent), 1/2 tsp.	0
Flax seeds:	
(Arrowhead Mills), 2 oz.	6.0 d
Flounder*	0
Flour, see "Wheat flour" and specific listings	
Fluke*	0
Frankfurter:	
meat or with cheese, 4 oz.	0
French toast, frozen:	
1 oz.	.8 d
1 medium piece, approximately 2.1 oz.	1.7 d
sticks *(Qwik-Krisp),* 4 pieces	1.0 d
French toast breakfast, vegetarian:	
frozen, cinnamon swirl, with patty *(Morningstar Farms),* 6.5 oz.	4.0 d
Frog's legs*	0

Frosting, ready-to-use:

chocolate, creamy, 1/12 can or package . . . .   .1 d

coconut, 1/12 can or package . . . .   1.0 d

cream cheese flavor, 1/12 can or package . . . .   .2 d

vanilla, creamy, 1/12 can or package . . . .   .1 d

Frosting mix:

all varieties *(Betty Crocker),* 1/12 mix . . . .   (0)

Fructose:

all varieties, 4 oz.   0

Fruit, see specific listings

Fruit, mixed, canned (see also "Fruit cocktail"
    and "Fruit salad"):

in juice *(Del Monte* Fruit Naturals), 1/2 cup . . . . . .   1.0 d

in extra light syrup *(Del Monte* Lite), 1/2 cup . . . . .   1.0 d

in heavy syrup *(Del Monte),* 1/2 cup . . . .   1.0 d

Fruit, mixed, frozen:

(Stilwell), 1 1/4 cup . . . .   1.0 d

sweetened[1], thawed, 5 oz. . . . .   2.7 d

in syrup *(Birds Eye),* 5 oz. . . . .   1.0 d

Fruit cocktail, canned:

(Hunt's), 4 oz. . . . .   <1.0 d

in juice, syrup, or water, 4 oz. . . . .   1.3 d

in water, 1/2 cup . . . .   1.3 d

in light syrup, 1/2 cup . . . .   1.4 d

Fruit-flavored soda:

carbonated, all varieties   0

Fruit juice, see specific fruit listings

Fruit punch juice drink:

bottled, 6 fl. oz. . . . .   (0)

frozen concentrate, undiluted, 6-fl.-oz. can . . . . . .   .4 d

Fruit punch drink:

bottled, 6 fl. oz. . . . .   .2 d

mix, 2 rounded tsp. . . . .   <.1 d

---

[1] Includes peaches, cherries, raspberries, boysenberries, and grapes.

Fruit salad, canned:
in heavy syrup, 4 oz. . . . .   1.3 d
in heavy syrup, 1/2 cup . . . .   1.4 d
tropical, in heavy syrup, 1/2 cup . . . .   1.7 d
Fudge, see "Candy"
Fudge topping, see "Chocolate topping"
Fuyu, see "Tofu"

G

Garbanzos, see "Chickpeas"
Garlic:
untrimmed, 1 lb. . . . . 8.3 d
trimmed, 1 oz. . . . . .6 d
1 clove, approximately .1 oz. untrimmed . . . . .1 d
Garlic pepper:
(*Lawry's* Spice Blends), 1 tsp. . . . . .1 c
Garlic powder:
1 oz. . . . . .5 d
1 tbsp. . . . . .1 d
1 tsp. . . . . <.1 d
with parsley (*Lawry's* Spice Blends), 1 tsp. . . . . . . .1 c
Garlic puree:
(*Progresso*), 1 tsp. 0
Garlic salt:
(*Lawry's* Spice Blends), 1 tsp. . . . . <.1 c
Garlic spread:
(*Lawry's*), ½ tbsp. . . . . <.1 c
concentrate (*Lawry's*), ½ tbsp. 0
Gefilte fish:
(*Mothers* Low Sodium), 1 piece . . . . <1.0 d
(*Rokeach*, 4 pieces), 1 piece . . . . 1.0 d
(*Rokeach*, 8 pieces), 1 piece 0
(*Rokeach* Low Sodium/No Sugar/Old Vienna),
1 piece . . . . 1.0 d

jelled broth:
    (Mothers Old Fashioned, 4 pieces), 1 piece . . .   1.0 d
    (Mothers Old Fashioned, 6 pieces), 1 piece . . .   2.0 d
    (Rokeach), 1 piece   0
    sweet *(Mothers* Old World), 1 piece . . . .   1.0 d
liquid broth *(Mothers* Old Fashioned), 1 piece . . .   1.0 d
sweet *(Rokeach* Gold Label/Old Vienna),
    1 piece . . . .   1.0 d
whitefish, jelled broth *(Rokeach* No Sugar),
    1 piece . . . .   1.0 d
whitefish/pike, jelled broth:
    (Mothers, 4 pieces), 1 piece . . . .   1.0 d
    (Rokeach), 1 piece . . . .   3.0 d
    (Rokeach Old Vienna), 1 piece . . . .   1.0 d
Gelatin, unflavored:
(Knox), 1 packet   0
Gelatin bar, frozen:
all flavors *(Jell-O Gelatin Pops),* 1 bar   0
Gelatin dessert:
(Jell-O Snacks), 3.5-oz. cup   0
mix, prepared, all flavors *(Jell-O),* ½ cup   0
Gin:
plain or flavored   0
Gingerroot:
untrimmed, 1 lb. . . . .   8.4 d
trimmed, 1 oz. . . . .   .6 d
sliced, ¼ cup . . . .   .5 d
Ginger, ground:
1 oz. . . . .   3.5 d
1 tsp. . . . .   .2 d
Ginkgo nuts:
shelled, raw, 1 oz. . . . .   .1 c
Ginkgo nuts, canned:
drained, 1 oz. . . . .   2.6 d
drained, ½ cup . . . .   7.2 d

Ginkgo nuts, dried, 1 oz. . . . . .3 c
Goat* 0
Godfather's Pizza:
original crust cheese, jumbo, ¹⁄₁₀ pie . . . . .7 d
original crust combo, jumbo, ¹⁄₁₀ pie . . . . 2.5 d
original crust pepperoni:
  mini, ¹⁄₄ pie . . . . .2 d
  small, ¹⁄₆ pie . . . . .5 d
  medium, ¹⁄₈ pie . . . . .5 d
  large, ¹⁄₁₀ pie . . . . .5 d
  jumbo, ¹⁄₁₀ pie . . . . .7 d
golden crust cheese or pepperoni:
  small, ¹⁄₆ pie . . . . .4 d
  medium, ¹⁄₈ pie . . . . .4 d
  large, ¹⁄₁₀ pie . . . . .5 d
Goose* 0
Goose liver* 0
Goose liver pâté:
canned, 4 oz. 0
Gooseberries, fresh:
trimmed, 4 oz. . . . . 4.9 d
trimmed, ½ cup . . . . 3.2 d
Gooseberries, canned:
in light syrup, 4 oz. . . . . 2.7 d
in light syrup, ½ cup . . . . 3.0 d
Gooseberries, Chinese, see "Kiwifruit"
Gourd, see specific listings
Gourd, dried, see "Kanpyo"
Grain, see specific listings
Grain entree mix, prepared:
3-grain, with herbs *(Quick Pilaf),* ½ cup . . . . 1.3 d
Granadilla, see "Passion fruit"
Granola, see "Cereal"

Granola and cereal bars (see also "Snack bars"):

all varieties (*Kellogg's Nutri·Grain*), 1 bar . . . . . . 1.0 d

all varieties, except raisin (*Health Valley* Fat Free), 1 bar . . . . 3.7 d

apple cinnamon or honey nut (*Nature Valley Granola Bites*), 1 pouch . . . . 2.0 d

chocolate chip or crunch (*Carnation* Breakfast), 1 bar . . . . .2 d

cinnamon (*Nature Valley*), 1 bar . . . . 1.0 d

oat bran–honey graham or oats 'n honey (*Nature Valley*), 1 bar . . . . 1.0 d

peanut butter (*Nature Valley*), 1 bar . . . . 1.0 d

peanut butter chocolate chip (*Carnation* Breakfast Bar), 1 bar . . . . .1 d

peanut butter crunch (*Carnation* Breakfast Bar), 1 bar 0

raisin (*Health Valley* Fat Free), 1 bar . . . . 3.0 d

Grape drink or soda:

bottled, 6 fl. oz. 0

Grape juice:

canned, bottled, or frozen and diluted, 6 fl. oz. . . .2 d

frozen concentrate, undiluted, 6 fl. oz. . . . . .6 d

Grape juice drink:

or cocktail, 6 fl. oz. .2 d

Grape leaf, in jars:

imported (*Krinos*), 1 oz. . . . . 2.0 d

Grapes, fresh:

American type (slipskin):

with seeds, 1 lb. . . . . 5.0 d

10 medium, approximately 1.4 oz. with seeds . . .3 d

peeled and seeded, 1/2 cup . . . . .6 d

European type (adherent skin):

seedless or seeded, 1 lb. . . . . 2.7 d

seedless, 10 medium, approximately 1¾ oz. . . .3 d

seedless or seeded, 1/2 cup . . . . .5 d

Grapes, canned (Thompson seedless):

in water, 4 oz. . . . .   1.1 d

in water, ½ cup . . . .   1.2 d

in heavy syrup, 4 oz.   .5 d

in heavy syrup, ½ cup . . . .   .5 d

Grape-fruit juice drink:

or cocktail, 6 fl. oz. . . . .   (0)

Grapefruit, fresh:

all varieties, untrimmed, 1 lb. . . . .   2.5 d

pink or red, ½ medium, 3¾″ diameter,

   approximately 8.5 oz. . . . .   1.4 d

pink or red, sections with juice, ½ cup . . . .   1.3 c

white, ½ medium, 3¾″ diameter, approximately

   8.5 oz. . . . .   1.3 d

white, ½ cup sections with juice . . . .   1.3 d

Grapefruit, canned, or chilled:

in juice, syrup, or water, 4 oz. or ½ cup . . . .   .5 d

Grapefruit juice:

fresh, 6 fl. oz. or juice from 1 medium white

   grapefruit . . . .   .2 d

canned, bottled, or frozen and diluted, 6 fl. oz.   . .   .2 d

frozen concentrate, undiluted, 6 fl. oz. . . . .   .8 d

Grapefruit juice drink:

or cocktail, 6 fl. oz. . . . .   .2 d

Grapeseed oil:

all varieties   0

Gravy, see specific listings

Great northern beans, dry:

uncooked, 1 oz. . . . .   11.3 d

uncooked, ½ cup . . . .   36.4 d

boiled, ½ cup . . . .   6.2 d

Great northern beans, canned:

with liquid, 4 oz. . . . .   5.6 d

with liquid, ½ cup . . . .   6.4 d

(Allens), ½ cup . . . .   5.0 d

(Eden), ½ cup . . . .   6.4 d

(Green Giant/Joan of Arc), ½ cup	5.0 d
(Hain), 4 oz.	7.0 d

Green beans, fresh:

raw:

untrimmed, 1 lb.	13.6 d
trimmed, 4 oz.	3.9 d
trimmed, ½ cup	1.9 d
boiled, drained, ½ cup	2.0 d

Green beans, canned, or packaged:

with liquid, 4 oz. or ½ cup	.8 d
drained, 4 oz.	2.2 d
drained, ½ cup	1.3 d
(Green Giant Kitchen Sliced), ½ cup	1.0 d
cut or French *(Green Giant/Green Giant Pantry Express)*, ½ cup	1.0 d
almondine *(Green Giant)*, ½ cup	2.0 d
seasoned, ½ cup	1.0 c

Green beans, frozen:

unheated, 3.3 oz.	2.7 d
boiled, drained, ½ cup	2.2 d
(Green Giant/Green Giant Harvest Fresh), ½ cup	1.0 d
in butter sauce *(Green Giant One Serving)*, 5.5. oz.	3.0 d
in butter sauce, cut *(Green Giant)*, ½ cup	1.5 d
French, with toasted almonds *(Birds Eye)*, 3 oz. .	2.0 d

Green bean combinations, frozen or packaged:

mushroom, creamy *(Green Giant Garden Gourmet Right for Lunch)*, 9.5 oz.	4.0 d
potatoes and mushrooms, in sauce *(Green Giant Pantry Express)*, ½ cup	2.5 d

Green peas, sweet, fresh:

raw:

in pod, untrimmed, 1 lb.	8.8 d

Green peas, raw *(cont.)*
shelled, 4 oz. . . . .   5.8 d
shelled, ½ cup . . . .   3.7 d
boiled, drained, ½ cup . . . .   4.4 d
Green peas, canned:
with liquid, 4 oz. . . . .   2.2 d
with liquid, ½ cup . . . .   2.4 d
drained, 4 oz. . . . .   4.6 d
drained, ½ cup . . . .   3.5 d
dry early June *(Crest Top),* ½ cup . . . .   5.0 d
sweet *(Green Giant 50% Less Salt),* ½ cup . . . . .   3.0 d
very young, early, small *(Green Giant),* ½ cup . . .   3.0 d
very young, sweet, small or tender *(Green
    Giant),* ½ cup . . . .   4.0 d
Green peas, frozen:
unheated, 3.3 oz. . . . .   4.4 d
boiled, drained, ½ cup . . . .   4.4 d
early, baby, *Le Sueur (Green Giant Harvest
    Fresh),* ½ cup . . . .   3.0 d
early, baby, *Le Sueur (Green Giant* Select),
    ½ cup . . . .   4.0 d
sweet *(Green Giant),* ½ cup . . . .   4.0 d
sweet *(Green Giant Harvest Fresh),* ½ cup . . . . .   3.0 d
in butter sauce:
    early, baby, *Le Sueur (Green Giant),* ½ cup . . .   3.0 d
    early, baby, *Le Sueur (Green Giant* One
        Serving), 4.5 oz. . . . .   5.0 d
    sweet *(Green Giant),* ½ cup . . . .   4.0 d
    sweet, tender *(Birds Eye),* ½ cup . . . .   3.0 d
Le Sueur style *(Green Giant Valley
    Combinations),* ½ cup . . . .   2.0 d
Green peas, dried, see "Split peas"
Green pepper, see "Pepper, sweet"
Grenadine syrup:
(Rose's), 1 tbsp.   0
Grits, see "Corn grits"

Ground cherries:
trimmed, 1/2 cup . . . . 2.0 c
Grouper* 0
Guacamole seasoning:
(Lawry's Seasoning Blends), 1 package . . . . .8 c
mix *(Old El Paso),* 1/7 package 0
Guava:
untrimmed, 1 lb. . . . . 19.6 d
1 medium, approximately 4 oz. untrimmed . . . . . 4.9 d
1/2 cup . . . . 4.5 d
Guava fruit drink:
(Ocean Spray Mauna La'I), 6 fl. oz. . . . . (0)
Guava sauce:
cooked, 1/2 cup . . . . 4.3 d
Guava–passion fruit drink:
(Ocean Spray Mauna La'I), 6 fl. oz. . . . . (0)
Guinea hen* 0
Gumbo dinner mix:
(Luzianne), 1/5 package . . . . 1.0 d

H

Food and Measure	Fiber Grams

Haddock* 0
Hake* 0
Halibut* 0
Ham* 0
Ham salad spread:
(Libby's Spreadables), 1.9 oz. . . . . .6 d
Ham spread, deviled:
(Hormel), 1 oz. 0
(Underwood), 2⅛ oz. 0
Hamburger patty:
all meat 0
"Hamburger," vegetarian, mix, prepared:
(Nature's Burger), 3 oz. . . . . 4.0 d
burger *(Tofu Classics)*, 3.4 oz. . . . . 2.6 d
BBQ or pizza flavor *(Nature's Burger)*, 3 oz. . . . . 3.0 d
Hazelnut oil:
all varieties 0
Hazelnuts:
dried, unblanched:
  in shell, 1 lb. . . . . 12.7 d
  shelled, 1 oz. . . . . 1.7 d
  whole, ½ cup . . . . 4.1 d
  chopped, ½ cup . . . . 7.5 d
  ground, ½ cup . . . . 2.3 d
dry-roasted, 1 oz. . . . . 1.1 d

oil-roasted, 1 oz. . . . . 1.8 d
Head cheese:
all varieties, 4 oz. 0
Heart* 0
Herb garlic marinade:
with lemon juice *(Lawry's)*, 2 tbsp. . . . . .4 c
Herbs, see specific listings
Herbs, mixed:
(Lawry's Pinch of Herbs), 1 tsp. . . . . .2 c
Herring* 0
Herring, pickled:
Cajun *(Elf)*, 3 oz. 0
in cream or wine sauce *(Elf)*, 3 oz. 0
in dill, horseradish, or cocktail sauce *(Elf)*, 4 oz. 0
rollmops *(Elf)*, 3 oz. 0
Herring oil:
all varieties 0
Hickory nuts, dried:
in shell, 1 lb. . . . . 9.3 d
shelled, 1 oz. . . . . 1.8 d
Hollandaise sauce:
½ cup 0
Hominy, canned (see also "Corn grits"):
white or yellow, 4 oz. 2.9 d
white or yellow, ½ cup . . . . 2.0 d
Honey:
2 oz. . . . . <.1 d
Honey bun, see "Buns, sweet" and "Rolls,
   sweet"
Honey butter:
(Honey Butter), 1 tbsp. 0
Honey loaf:
all varieties 0
Honey roll sausage:
all varieties 0

Honeycomb:
strained *(Frieda's)*, 1 oz. 0
Honeydew:
untrimmed, 1 lb. . . . . 1.3 d
2″ slice, ¹/₁₀ of 7″ melon, approximately 8 oz.
   untrimmed . . . . .8 d
pulp, cubed, ½ cup . . . . .5 d
Horseradish-tree, fresh:
leafy tips:
   raw, untrimmed, 1 lb. . . . . 5.6 d
   raw, chopped, ½ cup . . . . .2 d
   boiled, drained, chopped, ½ cup . . . . .4 d
pods:
   raw, untrimmed, 1 lb. . . . . 7.6 d
   raw, sliced, ½ cup . . . . 1.6 d
   boiled, drained, sliced, ½ cup . . . . 2.5 d
Hot dog:
all meat or with cheese, 4 oz. 0
Hot sauce, see "Pepper sauce, hot" and
   specific listings
Hubbard squash:
raw, untrimmed, 1 lb. . . . . 4.4 d
raw, cubed, ½ cup . . . . .9 d
baked, cubed, ½ cup . . . . 2.9 d
boiled, drained, mashed, ½ cup . . . . 3.4 d
Hummus:
1 oz. . . . . 1.4 d
¼ cup . . . . 3.1 d
1 tbsp. . . . . .1 d
Hummus mix:
prepared *(Fantastic Foods)*, ¼ cup . . . . 3.5 d
Hush puppies:
1 oz. . . . . .8 d
Hush puppies, frozen:
regular or jalapeño *(Stilwell)*, 3 pieces . . . . 2.0 d

Hyacinth beans, fresh:

raw, trimmed, 1/2 cup .5 c

boiled, drained, 1/2 cup . . . . .8 c

Hyacinth beans, mature, dry, boiled, 1/2 cup . . . 2.4 c

I

Food and Measure	Fiber Grams

Ice (see also "Sherbet"):
lemon or lime, ½ cup 0
Italian, chocolate *(MamaTish's)*, ½ cup . . . . 2.0 d
Italian, lemon, raspberry or strawberry
   (MamaTish's), ½ cup 0
Ice bar, frozen, fruit flavored, 3-fl.-oz. bar 0
Ice cream, vanilla, ½ cup 0
"Ice cream," substitute or imitation, ½ cup:
brownie chunk fudge swirl *(Simple Pleasures*
   Light), ½ cup . . . . 1.0 d
café au lait *(Edy's Grand Light)*, ½ cup 0
caramel *Brickle (Simple Pleasures* Light), ½ cup 0
chocolate, Dutch *(Simple Pleasures* Light),
   ½ cup . . . . 1.0 d
chocolate caramel *(C'est Bon Chocolat)*, ½ cup . 2.0 d
chocolate caramel sundae *(Simple Pleasures*
   Light), ½ cup . . . . 1.0 d
chocolate cherry/brandy *(C'est Bon Chocolat)*,
   ½ cup . . . . 2.0 d
chocolate chip:
   (Edy's Grand Light), ½ cup . . . . (0)
   (Edy's Sugar Free), ½ cup . . . . (0)
   (Healthy Choice), ½ cup . . . . (0)
   cherry, Bordeaux *(Healthy Choice)*, ½ cup . . . . . . (0)

cookie dough *(Simple Pleasures* Light),
   ½ cup   0
mint *(Healthy Choice),* ½ cup . . . .   (0)
chocolate fudge mousse *(Edy's Grand Light),*
   ½ cup . . . .   (0)
chocolate raspberry *(C'est Bon Chocolat),*
   ½ cup . . . .   2.0 d
coffee toffee *(Healthy Choice),* ½ cup   0
fudge *(Edy's Grand Light),* ½ cup . . . .   (0)
fudge, chocolate or marble *(Edy's* Fat Free),
   ½ cup . . . .   (0)
rocky road *(Simple Pleasures* Light), ½ cup . . . .   1.0 d
toffee crunch *(Simple Pleasures),* ½ cup   0
vanilla, ½ cup   0
vanilla 'n caramel *(Edy's* Sugar Free), ½ cup   0
vanilla fudge royale *(Sealtest Free),* ½ cup . . . .   (0)
vanilla fudge swirl *(Simple Pleasures* Light),
   ½ cup   0
vanilla-chocolate-strawberry *(Sealtest Free)* . . . .   (0)
vanilla-strawberry royale *(Sealtest Free)* . . . .   (0)
Ice cream cone or cup, unfilled:
cake or wafer type, 1 piece, approximately
   .1 oz. . . . .   .2 d
sugar cone, 1 piece, approximately .4 oz. . . . .   .5 d
Ice milk, vanilla, ½ cup   0
Icing, cake, see "Frosting"
Indian date, see "Tamarind"
Irish moss, see "Seaweed"
Italian chestnuts, see "Chestnuts, European"
Italian sausage:
all varieties, 4 oz.   0
Italian seasoning:
(Tone's), 1 tsp. . . . .   .2 d

J

Food and Measure	Fiber Grams

Jackfish* 0
Jackfruit:
untrimmed, 1 lb. . . . . 2.0 d
trimmed, 1 oz. . . . . .5 d
Jalapeño:
fresh, see "Pepper, chili"
canned, with liquid, 4 oz. . . . . 2.6 d
Jamaican jerk:
dipping sauce *(Helen's Tropical Exotics)*, 2 tbsp. . 1.0 d
seasoning and marinade *(Helen's Tropical
    Exotics)*, 1 tbsp. dry . . . . 1.0 d
Jambalaya dinner mix:
(Luzianne), ¼ package . . . . 1.0 d
Jams and preserves:
apricot *(Chambord)*, 1 tbsp. . . . . .2 d
black currant *(Chambord)*, 1 tbsp. . . . . .7 d
blueberry *(Chambord)*, 1 tbsp. . . . . .4 d
cherry, black *(Chambord)*, 1 tbsp. . . . . .2 d
four fruit *(Chambord)*, 1 tbsp. . . . . .5 d
orange *(Chambord)*, 1 tbsp. . . . . .4 d
orange marmalade, 1 tbsp. . . . . .1 d
peach *(Chambord)*, 1 tbsp. . . . . .2 d
plum *(Chambord* Fancy), 1 tbsp. . . . . .3 d
raspberry, black *(Chambord)*, 1 tbsp. . . . . .7 d

raspberry, red *(Chambord)*, 1 tbsp. . . . . .5 d
strawberry *(Chambord)*, 1 tbsp. . . . . .3 d
Java plum:
3 medium, .4 oz. . . . . <.1 c
seeded, ½ cup . . . . .2 c
Jelly, fruit:
all flavors, 1 oz. . . . . .3 d
all flavors, 1 tbsp. . . . . .1 d
Jerusalem artichoke:
raw, untrimmed, 1 lb. . . . . 5.0 d
trimmed, 4 oz. . . . . 1.8 d
trimmed, sliced, ½ cup . . . . 1.2 d
Jew's ear, raw:
untrimmed, 1 lb. . . . . 9.5 c
sliced, ½ cup . . . . 2.1 c
Jew's ear, dried:
1 oz. . . . . 8.8 c
½ cup . . . . 3.7 c
Jicama, see "Yam bean tuber"
Jujube:
raw, seeded, 1 oz. . . . . .4 c
dried, 1 oz. . . . . .9 c
Jute, potherb:
raw, untrimmed, 1 lb. . . . . 3.4 c
raw, ½ cup . . . . .2 c
boiled, drained, ½ cup . . . . .9 d

K

Food and Measure	Fiber Grams

Kale, fresh:

raw:

    untrimmed, 1 lb. .... 5.5 d

    trimmed, 4 oz. .... 2.3 d

    trimmed, chopped, ½ cup .... .7 d

boiled, drained, chopped, ½ cup .... 1.3 d

Kale, canned:

(Allens/Sunshine), ½ cup .... 2.0 d

Kale, frozen:

unheated, 3.3 oz., ⅓ of 10-oz. package ...... 2.0 d

Kale, Scotch:

raw, untrimmed, 1 lb. .... 3.4 c

raw, chopped, ½ cup .... .4 c

boiled, drained, chopped, ½ cup .... .6 c

Kamut:

flakes *(Arrowhead Mills),* 1 oz. .... 3.0 d

grain, rolled, or flour *(Arrowhead Mills),* 2 oz. .... 4.0 d

Kanpyo:

1 oz. .... 2.6 c

3 strips, approximately .7 oz. .... 1.7 c

½ cup .... 2.5 c

Kasha, see "Buckwheat groats"

Kelp, see "Seaweed"

Kidney beans, dry:

uncooked:

1 oz.	7.1 d
½ cup	22.9 d
(Arrowhead Mills), 2 oz.	11.7 d
boiled, ½ cup	6.5 d

Kidney beans, canned:

red:

with liquid, 4 oz.	7.3 d
with liquid, ½ cup	8.2 d
(Hunt's), 4 oz.	5.0 d
(Progresso), 4 oz.	7.0 d
dark *(Allens/East Texas Fair)*, ½ cup	6.0 d
dark *(Hain)*, 4 oz.	7.0 d
dark or light *(Green Giant/Joan of Arc)*, ½ cup	5.0 d
light *(Allens)*, ½ cup	6.0 d
white *(Progresso* Cannellini)*, 4 oz.	6.5 d

Kidneys* ... 0

Kielbasa:

all varieties, 4 oz. ... 0

Kingfish* ... 0

Kirsch:

plain or flavored ... 0

Kiwifruit, fresh:

untrimmed, 1 lb.	13.3 d
1 large, approximately 3.7 oz. untrimmed	3.1 d
1 medium, approximately 3.1 oz. untrimmed	2.6 d

Knockwurst:

all varieties, 4 oz. ... 0

Kohlrabi, fresh:

raw:

untrimmed, 1 lb.	7.5 d
trimmed, 4 oz.	4.1 d
trimmed, sliced, ½ cup	2.5 d
boiled, drained, sliced, ½ cup	.9 d

Koyadofu, see "Tofu"

Kumquat:

untrimmed, 1 lb. . . . . 27.9 d
1 medium, approximately ¾ oz. untrimmed . . . . 1.3 d
seeded, 4 oz. . . . . 7.5 d

L

Food and Measure	Fiber Grams

Lake herring*	0
Lake trout*	0
Lamb*	0
Lamb's-quarters:	
raw, 4 oz.	4.6 d
boiled, drained, chopped, ½ cup	1.9 d
Lard:	
pork	0
Lasagna entree, frozen:	
(Celentano), 10 oz.	7.0 d
(Celentano Great Choice), 10 oz.	2.0 d
primavera *(Celentano Great Choice),* 10 oz.	7.0 d
Lasagna sheets, see "Pasta," and "Pasta, frozen"	
Laver, see "Seaweed"	
Leeks, fresh:	
raw:	
untrimmed, 1 lb.	3.6 d
1 medium, approximately 9.9 oz. untrimmed	2.2 d
trimmed, chopped, ½ cup	.9 d
boiled, drained, chopped, ½ cup	.4 c
Leeks, freeze-dried, 1 tbsp.	<.1 c

Lemon, fresh:

pulp from 1 medium, 2⅛″ diameter,

   approximately 3.9 oz. untrimmed . . . . 1.6 d

pulp, 1 oz. . . . . .8 d

Lemon juice:

fresh, 1 fl. oz. or 2 tbsp. . . . . .1 d

Lemon peel:

peel from 1 medium lemon, approximately

   1.7 oz. . . . . 5.2 d

1 tbsp. . . . . .6 d

1 tsp. . . . . .2 d

Lemon pepper:

(Lawry's Spice Blends), 1 tsp. . . . . .1 c

Lemonade:

chilled or frozen and diluted, 8 fl. oz. . . . . (0)

frozen concentrate, undiluted, 6-fl.-oz. can . . . . . . .8 d

Lemonade flavor drink:

fluid or mix, 6 fl. oz. 0

Lentil dishes:

canned, hearty, with vegetables *(Health Valley*

   Fast Menu Fat Free), 5 oz. . . . . 10.3 d

mix, prepared:

   and couscous *(Fantastic Only a Pinch),* 10 oz. . 10.0 d

   curried, with rice *(Fantastic),* 10 oz. . . . . 8.0 d

   pilaf, with couscous *(Fantastic Leapin'*

     Lentils), 10 oz. . . . . 9.0 d

Lentils, dry:

uncooked:

   1 oz. . . . . 8.6 d

   ½ cup . . . . 29.3 d

   green or red *(Arrowhead Mills),* 2 oz. . . . . 8.8 d

boiled, ½ cup . . . . 7.8 d

Lentils, sprouted, raw:

2 oz. . . . . 2.0 c

½ cup . . . . 1.2 c

Lettuce, fresh:

bibb, Boston, or butterhead:

  untrimmed, 1 lb. 3.6 d

  1 head, 5" diameter, approximately 7.8 oz.

    untrimmed . . . . 1.6 d

  2 inner leaves, approximately ½ oz. . . . . .5 d

cos or romaine:

  untrimmed, 1 lb. 10.2 d

  1 inner leaf, approximately .3 oz. . . . . .2 d

  shredded, ½ cup . . . . .7 d

iceberg or crisphead:

  untrimmed, 1 lb. 6.0 d

  1 head, 6" diameter, approximately 1¼ lbs.

    untrimmed . . . . 7.5 d

  1 leaf, approximately .7 oz. . . . . .3 d

looseleaf:

  untrimmed, 1 lb. 5.5 d

  1 leaf, approximately .3 oz. . . . . .2 d

  shredded, ½ cup . . . . .5 d

Lima beans, immature, fresh:

raw, in pod, 1 lb. 9.8 d

raw, trimmed, ½ cup . . . . 3.8 d

boiled, drained, ½ cup . . . . 4.5 d

Lima beans, canned, immature:

with liquid, 4 oz. 3.6 d

with liquid, ½ cup . . . . 4.0 d

(*Green Giant/Joan of Arc* Butter Beans), ½ cup . 4.0 d

large (*Allens* Butterbeans), ½ cup . . . . 4.0 d

Lima beans, frozen, immature:

baby or Fordhook, unheated, 3.3 oz. . . . . 4.0 d

baby (*Green Giant Harvest Fresh*), ½ cup . . . . . 4.0 d

Fordhook, cooked, drained, ½ cup . . . . 6.1 d

in butter sauce (*Green Giant*), ½ cup . . . . 4.5 d

Lima beans, mature, dry:

uncooked:

  baby, 1 oz. . . . . 2.8 d

Lima beans, mature, uncooked *(cont.)*
baby, ½ cup . . . . 10.1 d
large, 1 oz. . . . . 5.4 d
large, ½ cup . . . . 16.9 d
boiled, baby, ½ cup . . . . 7.0 d
boiled, large, ½ cup . . . . 6.6 d
Lima beans, mature, canned:
with liquid, 4 oz. 5.5 d
with liquid, ½ cup . . . . 5.8 d
Lime, fresh:
untrimmed, 1 lb. 10.7 d
1 medium, 2″ diameter, approximately 2.8 oz.
untrimmed . . . . 1.9 d
pulp, 1 oz. . . . . .8 d
Lime juice:
fresh, 1 fl. oz. or 2 tbsp. . . . . .1 d
fresh, bottled, or frozen and diluted, 4 fl. oz. . . . . . .5 d
Limeade:
frozen concentrate, undiluted, 6-fl.-oz. can . . . . . . .8 d
key lime *(Boku),* 8 fl. oz. 0
Ling* 0
Ling cod* 0
Linguine, see "Pasta"
Liquor, pure distilled:
all varieties and blends 0
Litchi nuts, see "Lychees"
Little Caesars, 1 serving:
Crazy Bread, 1 piece . . . . 1.0 d
Crazy Sauce . . . . 4.0 d
Pizza! Pizza!, cheese or cheese and pepperoni,
1 slice:
round, small . . . . 2.0 d
round, medium or large . . . . 3.0 d
square, small, medium or large . . . . 3.0 d
salads:
antipasto, small . . . . 2.0 d

Greek, small . . . .   1.0 d
tossed, small. . . . .   2.0 d
sandwiches:
  ham and cheese or Italian . . . .   4.0 d
  tuna . . . .   6.0 d
  turkey . . . .   3.0 d
  veggie . . . .   4.0 d
Liver*   0
Liver cheese lunchon meat:
all varieties, 4 oz.   0
Liver pâté, see "Chicken liver pâté" and
  "Goose liver pâté"
Liver sausage or liverwurst:
all varieties, 4 oz.   0
Lobster*   0
"Lobster," imitation:
made from surimi   0
(Louis Kemp Lobster Delights), 2 oz.   0
Lobster sauce, rock:
canned (Progresso), ½ cup . . . .   2.0 d
Loganberries, fresh:
½ cup . . . .   2.2 c
Loganberries, frozen:
5 oz. . . . .   6.9 d
½ cup . . . .   3.6 d
Long rice, see "Noodles, Chinese"
Longan:
untrimmed, 1 lb. . . . .   2.6 d
10 medium, approximately 2.1 oz. untrimmed . . . .   .3 d
shelled and seeded, 1 oz. . . . .   .3 d
Longan, dried, 1 oz. . . . .   .6 c
Loquat:
untrimmed, 1 lb. . . . .   4.8 d
10 medium, approximately 5.6 oz. untrimmed . . .   1.7 d
peeled and seeded, 1 oz. . . . .   .5 d
Lotte*   0

Lotus root:
raw, untrimmed, 1 lb. . . . . 17.6 d
raw, trimmed, 1 oz. 1.4 d
boiled, drained, 10 slices, approximately 3.1 oz. . 2.8 d
boiled, drained, 4 oz. . . . . 3.5 d
Lotus seeds:
raw, 1 oz. . . . . .2 c
dried, 1 oz. . . . . .7 c
fried, 1 cup . . . . .8 c
Lox:
all varieties 0
Lunch combinations:
all meat and poultry varieties, except
    spreadables *(Lunchables),* 1 pkg. . . . . 1.0 d
spreadable, ham, garden vegetable or herb and
    chive *(Lunchables),* 1 pkg. . . . . <1.0 d
spreadable, turkey, green onion or ranch and
    herb *(Lunchables),* 1 pkg. . . . . 2.0 d
Luncheon meat, see specific listings
Lupins, dry:
uncooked, 1 oz. . . . . 3.9 c
uncooked, ½ cup . . . . 12.4 c
boiled, ½ cup . . . . 2.3 d
Lychees, fresh:
untrimmed, 1 lb. . . . . 3.5 d
10 medium, approximately 5.6 oz. untrimmed . . . 1.2 d
seeded, ½ cup . . . . 1.2 d
seeded, 1 oz. . . . . .4 d
Lychees, dried:
1 oz. . . . . 1.3 d

M

Macadamia nuts, dried:
shelled, 1 oz.	2.6 d
dried, 1 cup	12.5 d
oil-roasted, 1 oz.	.5 c

Macaroni (see also "Pasta"):

uncooked:
2 oz.	1.4 d
protein fortified, 2 oz.	2.4 d
vegetable or tricolor, 2 oz.	2.4 d
whole wheat, 2 oz.	2.4 d
elbow, ½ cup	1.3 d

cooked, elbow:
½ cup	1.1 d
vegetable or tricolor, 4 oz.	4.9 d
whole wheat, ½ cup	3.1 d

Macaroni and cheese:
frozen (Green Giant One Serving), 5.7 oz.	1.5 d

Macaroni and cheese mix, prepared:
regular or Parmesan (Fantastic Foods), ½ cup	2.6 d

Macaroni entree:

small, with tomato sauce (Mothers Choice),
7.5 oz.	1.0 d

Mace, ground:
1 oz.	5.7 d
1 tsp.	.3 d

Mackerel* 0
Mahimahi* 0
Mai tai cocktail mixer:
bottled *(Holland House),* 4.5 fl. oz. . . . . (0)
Malt cooler:
all varieties *(Bartles & Jaymes),* 6 fl. oz. 0
Malted milk flavor mix:
chocolate, 3 heaping tsp. . . . . .2 d
natural, 3 heaping tsp. . . . . .1 d
Mammy apple:
untrimmed, 1 lb. . . . . 8.2 d
½ medium, approximately 1.5 lbs. untrimmed . . . 12.7 d
peeled and seeded, 1 oz. . . . . .9 d
Mandarin orange, see "Tangerine"
Mango:
untrimmed, 1 lb. . . . . 5.6 d
1 medium, approximately 10.6 oz. untrimmed . . . 3.7 d
peeled, 1 oz. . . . . .5 d
peeled, sliced, ½ cup . . . . 1.5 d
Mango juice drink:
bottled, 6 fl. oz. . . . . (0)
Manhattan cocktail mixer:
bottled *(Holland House),* 1 fl. oz. 0
Manicotti, stuffed:
frozen *(Celentano),* 7 oz. . . . . 7.0 d
Manicotti entree, frozen:
(Celentano Great Choice), 10 oz. . . . . 3.0 d
Florentine *(Celentano* Great Choice), 10 oz. . . . . . . 5.0 d
with sauce *(Celentano),* 10 oz. . . . . 9.0 d
Maple syrup:
natural or imitation, 4 fl. oz. 0
Margarine:
all varieties and blends 0

Margarita cocktail mixer:

bottled, regular or strawberry *(Holland House)*,
  3 fl. oz. . . . . (0)

frozen, prepared with liquor *(Bacardi)*, 7 fl. oz. . . . . . (0)

Marinade, see specific listings

Marjoram, dried:

1 oz. . . . . 5.1 d

1 tsp. . . . . .1 d

Marmalade, see "Jams and preserves"

Marrow squash:

raw, trimmed, 1 oz. . . . . .1 c

Marshmallow topping:

(Smucker's), 2 tbsp. 0

plain or raspberry *(Marshmallow Fluff)*,
  1 heaping tsp. 0

Matzo, see "Crackers"

Matzo crumbs:

(Manischewitz Farfel), 1 cup . . . . .2 d

Matzo meal:

(Manischewitz Daily), 1 cup . . . . .5 d

Mayonnaise:

all varieties and blends, 2 tbsp. 0

Meat* 0

Meat, potted:

all varieties 0

Meat loaf seasoning mix:

(Lawry's Seasoning Blends), 1 package . . . . 1.8 c

Meat tenderizer:

unseasoned *(Tone's)*, 1 tsp. . . . . tr. d

Melon, see specific listings

Melon balls, frozen:

cantaloupe and honeydew, 5 oz. . . . . 1.0 d

cantaloupe and honeydew, ½ cup . . . . .6 d

Menudo seasoning mix:

(Gebhardt), 1 tsp. <1.0 d

Mesquite marinade:

(Lawry's), 2 tbsp. . . . . .1 c

Mexican beans, canned:

(Allens/Brown Beauty), ½ cup . . . . 5.0 d

(Old El Paso Mexe-Beans), ½ cup . . . . 13.0 d

Mexican seasoning:

(Tone's), 1 tsp. . . . . .4 d

rice *(Lawry's Seasoning Blends)*, 1 package . . . . 2.1 c

Milk, fluid:

dairy, all varieties 0

Milk, canned:

condensed or evaporated 0

Milk, chocolate, see "Chocolate drink or milk"

Milk, dry:

all varieties, 1 cup 0

"Milk," imitation, see "Soy milk"

Milk beverage, see specific listings

Milkfish* 0

Milkshake, frozen:

chocolate *(Micro-Magic)*, 1 shake . . . . (0)

Millet, dry:

uncooked:

   2 oz. . . . . 4.8 d

   ½ cup . . . . 8.5 d

   hulled *(Arrowhead Mills)*, 1 oz. . . . . 1.8 d

cooked, ½ cup . . . . 1.6 d

Millet flour:

(Arrowhead Mills), 2 oz. . . . . 3.7 d

Miso:

1 oz. . . . . 1.5 d

½ cup . . . . 7.6 d

Molasses:

all varieties, 4 fl. oz. 0

Monkfish* 0

Monosodium glutamate:

(Tone's), 1 tsp. 0

Mortadella:

all varieties, 4 oz. 0

Mothbeans:

boiled, 4 oz. . . . . 1.5 c

Mother's loaf:

pork, 1 oz. . . . . (0)

Mountain yam, Hawaiian:

raw, untrimmed, 1 lb. . . . . 1.7 c

raw, cubed, ½ cup . . . . .3 c

steamed, cubed, ½ cup . . . . .4 c

Muffins:

(Arnold Bran'nola), 1 piece . . . . 2.0 d

(Arnold Extra Crisp), 1 piece . . . . 1.0 d

apple:

  (Awrey's), 1.5 oz. piece 0

  spice *(Health Valley),* 1 piece . . . . 5.1 d

  streusel *(Awrey's),* 1 piece . . . . 1.0 d

  streusel *(Hostess* 97% Fat Free), 1 piece . . . . . 1.0 d

banana:

  (Health Valley), 1 piece . . . . 4.5 d

  nut *(Awrey's* Grande), 1 piece . . . . 1.0 d

  walnut, mini *(Hostess),* 5 pieces . . . . .6 d

blueberry:

  (Awrey's), 1.5-oz. piece . . . . 1.0 d

  (Awrey's Grande), 1 piece . . . . 2.0 d

  (Hostess 97% Fat Free), 1 piece . . . . 1.0 d

  apple *(Health Valley* Twin Pack), 1 piece . . . . . 5.0 d

  mini *(Hostess),* 5 pieces . . . . .7 d

carrot *(Health Valley* Twin Pack), 1 piece . . . . . . 5.0 d

cranberry or corn *(Awrey's),* 1 piece 0

English:

  (Roman Meal), 1 piece . . . . 2.5 d

  (Thomas'), 1 piece . . . . 1.0 d

  (Wonder Rounds), 1 piece . . . . 1.5 d

Muffins, English *(cont.)*

bran nut *(Thomas')*, 1 piece . . . .   4.0 d

cinnamon raisin *(Oatmeal Goodness)*, 1 piece .   2.1 d

cinnamon-raisin bran *(Pepperidge Farm*
  Wholesome Choice), 1 piece . . . .   4.0 d

honey & oatmeal *(Oatmeal Goodness)*,
  1 piece . . . .   1.6 d

honey wheat *(Thomas')*, 1 piece . . . .   3.0 d

oat bran *(Thomas', 12 pack)*, 1 piece . . . .   3.0 d

onion or raisin *(Thomas')*, 1 piece . . . .   2.0 d

raisin or sourdough *(Wonder* Rounds),
  1 piece . . . .   1.6 d

rye *(Thomas')*, 1 piece . . . .   3.0 d

sandwich size *(Thomas')*, 1 piece . . . .   2.0 d

sourdough *(Thomas')*, 1 piece . . . .   2.0 d

white, country *(Pepperidge Farm* Wholesome
  Choice), 1 piece . . . .   2.0 d

oat bran:

(Hostess), 1 piece . . . .   1.5 d

almond date *(Health Valley* Fancy Fruit),
  1 piece . . . .   8.2 d

banana nut *(Hostess)*, 1 piece . . . .   1.0 d

blueberry *(Health Valley* Fancy Fruit), 1 piece .   7.5 d

raisin *(Health Valley* Fancy Fruit), 1 piece . . . . .   7.7 d

raisin:

(Arnold), 1 piece . . . .   2.0 d

bran *(Awrey's)*, 1.5 oz. piece . . . .   1.0 d

bran *(Awrey's* Grande), 1 piece . . . .   3.0 d

raspberry *(Health Valley* Twin Pack), 1 piece . . . .   5.0 d

sourdough *(Arnold)*, 1 piece . . . .   1.0 d

Muffins, frozen or refrigerated:

apple oatmeal *(Pepperidge Farm* Wholesome
  Choice), 1 piece . . . .   3.0 d

blueberry *(Pepperidge Farm* Wholesome
  Choice), 1 piece . . . .   2.0 d

corn (*Pepperidge Farm* Wholesome Choice),
1 piece . . . .   1.0 d
English (*Roman Meal*), 1 piece . . . .   2.6 d
English, honey-nut oat bran (*Roman Meal*),
1 piece . . . .   2.2 d
raisin bran (*Pepperidge Farm* Wholesome
Choice), 1 piece . . . .   4.0 d

Muffin mix, prepared:
blueberry (*Arrowhead Mills* Blue), 1 piece . . . . . .   2.6 d
oat bran (*Arrowhead Mills* Wheat Free), 1 piece .   4.5 d
oat bran, apple spice (*Arrowhead Mills*), 1 piece .   5.4 d
wheat bran (*Arrowhead Mills*), 1 piece . . . . 10.5 d

Mulberries:
untrimmed, 1 lb. . . . .   7.7 d
10 berries, approximately ½ oz. . . . .   .3 d
½ cup . . . .   1.2 d

Mullet*   0

Mung beans, mature, dry:
uncooked:
   1 oz. . . . .   4.6 d
   ½ cup . . . . 17.0 d
   (*Arrowhead Mills*), 2 oz. . . . . 10.9 d
boiled, ½ cup . . . .   7.7 d

Mung beans, sprouted, fresh:
raw, 12-oz. package . . . .   6.1 d
raw, ½ cup . . . .   .9 d
boiled, ½ cup . . . .   .5 d

Mungo beans, dry:
raw, 1 oz. . . . .   1.3 c
boiled, ½ cup . . . .   5.8 d

Mushrooms, fresh:
raw:
   untrimmed, 1 lb.   5.3 d
   1 medium, approximately .7 oz. untrimmed . . . .   .2 d
   pieces, ½ cup . . . .   .4 d

Mushrooms *(cont.)*
boiled, 1 medium, approximately .4 oz. . . . .   .3 d
boiled, drained, pieces, ½ cup . . . .   1.7 d
Mushrooms, canned:
all cuts:
   drained, 4 oz. . . . .   2.7 d
   (Green Giant), ¼ cup . . . .   1.0 d
   plain or with garlic *(B in B)*, ¼ cup . . . .   1.0 d
drained, 1 medium, approximately .4 oz. . . . .   .3 d
drained, pieces, ½ cup . . . .   1.9 d
in butter sauce *(Green Giant)*, ½ cup . . . .   .6 d
Mushrooms, frozen:
whole *(Birds Eye* Deluxe), 2.6 oz. . . . .   2.0 d
battered *(Qwik-Krisp)*, 7 pieces . . . .   1.0 d
breaded *(Stilwell)*, 5 pieces . . . .   2.0 d
Mushrooms, oyster:
fresh *(Frieda's)*, 1 oz. . . . .   .2 d
Mushrooms, shiitake, fresh:
raw *(Frieda's)*, 1 oz. . . . .   .7 d
cooked, 4 medium or ½ cup pieces . . . .   1.5 d
Mushrooms, shiitake, dried:
1 oz. . . . .   3.3 d
1 medium, approximately .1 oz. . . . .   .4 d
Mushrooms, straw:
frozen *(Green Giant)*, ¼ cup . . . .   1.0 d
Muskellunge*   0
Mussels*   0
Mustard:
prepared, 1 tbsp.   0
Mustard greens, fresh:
raw, untrimmed, 1 lb. . . . .   8.4 d
raw, chopped, ½ cup, approximately 1 oz.
   untrimmed . . . .   .6 d
boiled, drained, chopped, ½ cup . . . .   1.4 d
Mustard greens, canned:
(Allens/Sunshine), ½ cup . . . .   1.0 d

Mustard greens, frozen, unheated:

chopped, 3.3 oz. . . . . 1.9 d

chopped, ½ cup . . . . 1.5 d

Mustard oil:

all varieties 0

Mustard powder:

(Spice Islands), 1 tsp. . . . . <.1 c

Mustard seeds, yellow:

1 oz. . . . . 1.9 d

1 tsp. . . . . .2 d

Mustard spinach:

raw, untrimmed, 1 lb. . . . . 4.2 c

raw, chopped, ½ cup . . . . .8 c

boiled, drained, chopped, ½ cup . . . . .7 c

Mutton* 0

N

Food and Measure	Fiber Grams

Nacho appetizer mix, regular or jalapeño:
(Tio Sancho Microwave Snacks):

chips, 4 oz.	4.0 c
cheese sauce, 3.5 oz.	.4 c

Natto:

1 oz.	1.5 d
½ cup	4.8 d

Navy beans, dry:

uncooked, 1 oz.	6.9 d
uncooked, ½ cup	25.4 d
boiled, ½ cup	3.3 d

Navy beans, canned:

(Allens), ½ cup	5.0 d
with liquid, 4 oz.	5.8 d
with liquid, ½ cup	6.7 d

Navy beans, sprouted:

raw, ½ cup	1.3 c
boiled, drained, 4 oz.	3.3 c

Neapolitan torte, see "Cake"

Nectarine:

untrimmed, 1 lb.	6.6 d
1 medium, 2½″ diameter, approximately 5.3 oz.	
untrimmed	2.2 d
sliced, ½ cup	1.1 d

New England Brand sausage:

all varieties, 4 oz. 0

New Zealand spinach:

raw, untrimmed, 1 lb. . . . . 2.3 c

raw, trimmed, 1 oz. or ½ cup chopped . . . . .2 c

boiled, drained, ½ cup . . . . .6 c

Newberg sauce, canned:

with sherry *(Snow's),* ⅓ cup 0

Noodles, Chinese:

cellophane or long rice, dry, 2 oz. . . . . <.1 c

chow mein:

  2 oz. . . . . 2.2 d

  ½ cup . . . . .9 d

  narrow or wide *(La Choy),* ½ cup . . . . <1.0 d

chow mein, wide *(La Choy),* ½ cup . . . . <1.0 d

rice *(La Choy),* ½ cup . . . . <1.0 d

Noodles, egg, dry:

uncooked, 2 oz. . . . . 1.5 d

uncooked, spinach, 2 oz. . . . . 3.9 d

cooked, ½ cup . . . . .9 d

cooked, spinach, ½ cup . . . . 1.8 d

Noodles, egg, frozen:

precooked *(Aunt Vi's),* 4 oz. . . . . 1.0 d

Noodles, Japanese:

somen, dry, 2 oz. . . . . 2.4 d

somen, cooked, 1 cup . . . . .4 c

Nutmeg, ground:

1 oz. . . . . 5.9 d

1 tsp. . . . . .5 d

Nuts, see specific listings

Nuts, mixed, 1 oz:

(Flavor House Deluxe), 1 oz. . . . . 2.0 d

with peanuts:

  dry-roasted, 1 oz. 2.6 d

  dry-roasted, ½ cup . . . . 6.2 d

Nuts, mixed, with peanuts *(cont.)*
   dry- or oil-roasted *(Flavor House),* 1 oz. . . . . . .   2.0 d
   oil-roasted, 1 oz.   2.8 d
   oil-roasted, ½ cup . . . .   7.0 d
"Nuts," wheat based, see "Wheat 'nuts' "

O

Food and Measure

Fiber Grams

Oat bran, raw:

1 oz. . . . . 4.5 d

½ cup . . . . 3.7 d

2 tbsp. . . . . .9 d

Oat flakes:

(Arrowhead Mills), 2 oz. . . . . 8.1 d

Oat flour:

(Arrowhead Mills), 2 oz. . . . . 8.3 d

Oat groats:

(Arrowhead Mills), 2 oz. . . . . 5.6 d

Oatmeal, see "Oats" and "Cereal"

Oats (see also "Cereal"), dry:

rolled or meal, 2 oz. . . . . 5.8 d

rolled or meal, ½ cup . . . . 4.2 d

steel cut *(Arrowhead Mills),* 2 oz. . . . . 2.8 d

Ocean perch* 0

Octopus* 0

Oheloberries:

untrimmed, 1 lb. . . . . 6.0 c

½ cup . . . . .9 c

Oil:

all varieties 0

Okara, see "Tofu"

Okra, fresh:

raw:

　untrimmed, 1 lb. 10.2 d

　8 pods, 3″ long, approximately 3.9 oz.

　　untrimmed . . . . 2.5 d

　　sliced, ½ cup . . . . 1.3 d

boiled, drained, 8 pods, 3″ long . . . . 2.1 d

boiled, drained, sliced, ½ cup . . . . 2.0 d

Okra, canned:

cut or with tomatoes *(Allens)*, ½ cup . . . . 2.0 d

Okra, frozen:

unheated, 3.3 oz. 2.1 d

boiled, drained, sliced, ½ cup . . . . 2.6 d

whole *(Stilwell)*, 9 pieces . . . . 4.0 d

cut *(Stilwell)*, ¾ cup or 3 oz. . . . . 3.0 d

breaded *(Stilwell Light)*, 21 pieces or 3 oz. . . . . . 1.0 d

Old-fashioned cocktail mixer:

bottled *(Holland House)*, 1 fl. oz. . . . . (0)

Old-fashioned loaf:

(Oscar Mayer), 1 slice 0

Olive loaf:

(Oscar Mayer), 1 slice 0

Olive oil:

all varieties 0

Olive salad:

(Progresso), ½ cup . . . . 2.0 d

Olives, pickled:

green, with pits:

　10 small . . . . .7 d

　10 large . . . . 1.0 d

　10 giant . . . . 1.7 d

green, pitted, 1 oz. .7 d

ripe, oil- or salt-cured, imported *(Krinos)*, ½ oz. 0

Onion, mature, fresh or stored:

raw:

　untrimmed, 1 lb. 7.4 d

trimmed, 1 oz. . . . . .5 d
chopped, 1/2 cup . . . . 1.4 d
chopped, 1 tbsp. .2 d
boiled, drained, chopped, 1/2 cup . . . . 1.5 d

Onion, canned:
with liquid, 4 oz. or 1/2 cup chopped . . . . 1.5 d
1 onion, 1" diameter, approximately 2.2 oz. . . . . . .8 d

Onion, frozen:
whole:
    unheated, 3.3 oz. . . . . 1.6 d
    boiled, drained, 2 oz. . . . . 1.3 d
    small *(Seabrook)*, 3.3 oz. . . . . 1.0 c
chopped, boiled, drained, 1 tbsp. . . . . .2 d
with cream sauce *(Birds Eye)*, 5 oz. . . . . 1.0 d
rings, see "Onion rings"

Onion, dried:
flakes, 1 tbsp. . . . . .5 d
minced *(Lawry's* Spice Blends), 1 tsp. . . . . .6 c

Onion, spring or green (scallion), with tops:
untrimmed, 1 lb. 11.3 d
trimmed, chopped, 1/2 cup . . . . 1.3 d
trimmed, chopped, 1 tbsp. . . . . .2 d

Onion, Welsh:
untrimmed, 1 lb. 3.0 c
trimmed, 1 oz. . . . . .3 c

Onion, wild, marinated:
(Krinos Volvi), 1 oz. . . . . 1.0 d

Onion flakes, see "Onion, dried"

Onion powder:
1 oz. . . . . 1.6 d
1 tsp. . . . . .1 d

Onion rings, frozen:
(Qwik-Krisp Natural Cut), 4 pieces . . . . 2.0 d
(Stilwell Crispy Crunchy), 6 pieces . . . . 5.0 d
beer battered *(Stilwell)*, 4 pieces . . . . 2.0 d

Onion rings *(cont.)*
breaded, par-fried, unheated, 3 oz., 1/3 of 9-oz.
  pkg. . . . . 1.1 d
Onion salt:
(Tone's), 1 tsp. . . . . <.1 d
Onion seeds, sprouted:
salad *(Shaw's* Premium), 2 oz. . . . . 3.0 d
Orange, fresh:
all varieties, untrimmed, 1 lb. . . . . 8.0 d
all varieties, pulp, 1 oz. . . . . .7 d
California:
  navel, 1 medium, 2^7/$_8$" diameter,
    approximately 7.2 oz. untrimmed . . . . 3.4 d
  navel, sections without membrane, 1/2 cup . . . . 2.0 d
  Valencia, 1 medium, 2^5/$_8$" diameter,
    approximately 5.7 oz. untrimmed . . . . 2.9 d
  Valencia, sections without membrane, 1/2 cup . 2.2 d
Florida, 1 medium, 2^{11}/$_{16}$" diameter,
  approximately 7.2 oz. . . . . 3.6 d
Florida, sections without membrane, 1/2 cup . . . . 2.2 d
Orange, canned, Mandarin, see "Tangerine"
Orange drink:
canned or bottled, 6 fl. oz. . . . . .2 d
breakfast, with pulp, frozen concentrate,
  undiluted, 6-fl.-oz. can . . . . .4 d
Orange juice:
fresh, juice from 2^5/$_8$"-diameter orange . . . . .2 d
fresh, canned, bottled, or frozen and diluted,
  6 fl. oz. . . . . .4 d
frozen concentrate, undiluted, 6 fl. oz. . . . . 1.7 d
Orange juice drink:
bottled, 6 fl. oz. . . . . (0)
Orange peel:
1 oz. . . . . 1.0 d
1 tbsp. . . . . .2 d

Orange sauce:
Mandarin *(La Choy),* 1 tbsp. . . . . .1 d
Orangeade:
bottled, 6 fl. oz. 0
Orange-apricot juice drink:
bottled, 6 fl. oz. . . . . .2 d
Orange-cranberry juice drink:
bottled, 6 fl. oz. . . . . .2 d
Orange-grapefruit juice:
bottled, 6 fl. oz. . . . . .2 d
Oregano, dried, ground:
1 oz. . . . . 4.3 d
1 tsp. . . . . .2 d
Oriental 5-spice:
(Tone's), 1 tsp. . . . . .5 d
Oyster* 0
Oyster plant, see "Salsify"
Oyster stew, see "Soup, canned, condensed"

P

P&B loaf:
(Kahn's), 1 slice 0
Palm oil:
all varieties 0
Pancake, frozen:
(Aunt Jemima Original), 3 pieces . . . . 1.5 d
(Hungry Jack Microwave Original), 3 pieces . . . . 2.0 d
blueberry or buttermilk (Hungry Jack
    Microwave), 3 pieces . . . . 1.0 d
oat bran or harvest wheat (Hungry Jack
    Microwave), 3 pieces . . . . 3.0 d
Pancake and waffle mix:
dry:
    complete, 1 oz. . . . . .8 d
    complete, ½ cup . . . . 1.6 d
    kamut (Arrowhead Mills), ¼ cup . . . . 4.0 d
    whole grain (Arrowhead Mills), ½ cup . . . . . . 10.0 d
    wild rice (Arrowhead Mills), 2½ oz. . . . . 4.3 d
prepared:
    (Hungry Jack Extra Lights), 3 pancakes,
        4″ each . . . . .5 d
    (Hungry Jack Extra Lights Complete),
        3 pancakes, 4″ each . . . . 1.0 d
    plain or buttermilk, complete, 4″ cake,
        approximately 1.3 oz. . . . . .5 d

plain or buttermilk, complete, 6" cake,
    approximately 2.7 oz. . . . . 1.0 d
  buckwheat, 3 pancakes, 4" each . . . . 2.1 d

Pancake syrup:
table blends, 4 fl. oz. 0

Pancreas* 0

Papaya:
1 medium, 3½" × 5⅛", approximately 1 lb.
    untrimmed . . . . 5.5 d
peeled and seeded, 1 oz. . . . . .5 d
peeled and seeded, cubed, ½ cup . . . . 1.3 d

Papaya nectar:
canned, 6 fl. oz. . . . . 1.1 d

Paprika:
1 oz. . . . . 5.9 d
1 tsp. . . . . .4 d

Parsley, fresh, raw:
untrimmed, 1 lb. . . . . 14.2 d
10 sprigs, approximately .4 oz. untrimmed . . . . . . .3 d
trimmed, chopped, ½ cup . . . . 1.0 d

Parsley, dried:
1 oz. . . . . 2.9 d
1 tsp. . . . . <.1 d

Parsley root:
1 oz. . . . . .4 d

Parsnip:
raw, untrimmed, 1 lb. . . . . 18.9 d
raw, sliced, ½ cup . . . . 3.3 d
boiled, drained, 1 medium, 9" × 2¼" diameter,
    approximately 5.6 oz. . . . . 6.4 d
boiled, drained, sliced, ½ cup . . . . 3.1 d

Passion fruit, purple:
untrimmed, 1 lb. . . . . 24.6 d
1 medium, approximately 1.2 oz. untrimmed . . . . 1.9 d
shelled, 1 oz. . . . . 2.9 d

Passion fruit juice, fresh:

purple or yellow, 6 fl. oz. . . . . .4 d

Pasta, dry (see also "Macaroni"):

uncooked[1]:

    regular, 2 oz. . . . . 1.4 d

    regular, spirals, 1/2 cup . . . . 1.0 d

    regular, small shells, 1/2 cup . . . . 1.1 d

    corn, 2 oz. . . . . 6.2 d

    protein fortified, 2 oz. . . . . 2.4 d

    protein fortified shells, 1/2 cup . . . . 2.0 d

    spinach, 2 oz. . . . . 6.0 d

    vegetable or tricolor, 2 oz. . . . . 2.4 d

    vegetable or tricolor spirals, 1/2 cup . . . . 1.8 d

    whole wheat, 2 oz. 7.0 d

cooked:

    regular, small shells, 1/2 cup . . . . 1.1 d

    regular, spaghetti, 1/2 cup . . . . 1.2 d

    regular, spirals, 1/2 cup . . . . 1.0 d

    corn spaghetti, 1/2 cup . . . . 3.4 d

    whole wheat spaghetti, 1/2 cup . . . . 3.1 d

Pasta, frozen, precooked:

regular, yolkless *(Aunt Vi's)*, 4 oz. . . . . 2.0 d

lasagna sheets *(Aunt Vi's)*, 4 oz. . . . . 2.0 d

Pasta dishes, frozen (see also specific pasta

  listings):

creamy cheddar *(Green Giant Pasta Accents),*

  1/2 cup . . . . 2.0 d

Dijon *(Green Giant Garden Gourmet Right for*

  Lunch), 9.5 oz. . . . . 4.0 d

garden herb seasoning *(Green Giant Pasta*

  Accents), 1/2 cup . . . . 3.0 d

garlic seasoning *(Green Giant Pasta Accents),*

  1/2 cup . . . . 2.0 d

[1] Includes all pasta forms and shapes—angel hair, bow ties, fettuccine, linguine, lasagna, rigatoni, penne, spaghetti, spirals, etc.—except as noted.

Florentine *(Green Giant Garden Gourmet Right for Lunch)*, 9.5 oz. . . . .   4.0 d
Parmesan, with sweet peas *(Green Giant One Serving)*, 5.5 oz.   2.5 d
primavera *(Green Giant Pasta Accents)*, ½ cup   .   2.5 d
Pasta dishes, mix (see also specific pasta listings), prepared:
cheese:
  cheddar, tangy *(Hain Pasta & Sauce)*, ½ cup   .   3.5 d
  Parmesan, creamy *(Hain Pasta & Sauce)*, ½ cup . . . .   3.0 d
  Swiss, creamy *(Hain Pasta & Sauce)*, ½ cup   .   3.5 d
dill, creamy, multibran *(Hain Pasta & Sauce)*, ½ cup . . . .   5.0 d
Italian, herb *(Hain Pasta & Sauce)*, ½ cup . . . . . .   4.0 d
Italian, multibran *(Hain Pasta & Sauce)*, ½ cup . . .   5.0 d
primavera *(Hain Pasta & Sauce)*, ½ cup . . . .   2.5 d
salad, Italian herb or spicy Oriental *(Fantastic)*, ½ cup . . . .   3.0 d
salsa, multibran *(Hain Pasta & Sauce)*, ½ cup . . .   5.0 d
Pasta and cheese, frozen:
baked *(Celentano)*, 10 oz. . . . .   8.0 d
Pasta salad, see "Pasta dishes, mix"
Pasta sauce (see also "Tomato sauce" and specific listings):
(Hunt's Chunky/Homestyle/Traditional), 4 oz. . . . .   2.0 d
(Pastorelli Italian Chef), 4 oz. . . . .   4.0 d
marinara *(Hain)*, 4 oz. . . . .   3.0 d
marinara *(Progresso)*, 4 oz. . . . .   <5.0 d
meat or meat flavor *(Hunt's/Hunt's Homestyle)*, 4 oz. . . . .   2.0 d
mushroom *(Hain)*, 4 oz. . . . .   3.0 d
mushroom *(Hunt's/Hunt's Homestyle)*, 4 oz. . . . .   2.0 d
Pasta sauce, refrigerated:
meatless *(Bodin's)*, 3.4 oz. . . . .   1.0 d

Pasta sauce mix:

(*Lawry's* Rich & Thick), 1 package . . . . .5 c

(*Spatini*), prepared, 1 cup . . . . <.1 c

with mushrooms (*Lawry's*), 1 package . . . . 2.1 c

Pastrami:

all varieties, 4 oz. 0

Pastry dough (see also "Pie crust shell"):

tart shell, 1 piece . . . . 2.0 d

Pâté, see specific listings

Pea pods, Chinese, see "Peas, edible-
  podded"

Peach, fresh:

untrimmed, 1 lb. . . . . 6.9 d

peeled, 1 medium, 2½″ diameter,

  approximately 4 per lb. untrimmed . . . . 1.7 d

peeled and pitted, 1 oz. . . . . .6 d

peeled and pitted, sliced, ½ cup . . . . 1.7 d

Peach, canned:

in juice, syrup, or water:

  4 oz. . . . . 1.1 d

  ½ cup . . . . 1.2 d

  1 peach half and 1⅔ tbsp. liquid . . . . .8 d

in juice, diced (*Del Monte* Fruit Naturals),

  ½ cup . . . . 1.0 d

in extra light syrup, diced (*Del Monte* Lite),

  ½ cup . . . . 1.0 d

in heavy syrup, diced (*Del Monte*), ½ cup . . . . . . 1.0 d

spiced, in syrup:

  4 oz. . . . . 1.1 d

  ½ cup . . . . 1.2 d

  1 peach and 2 tbsp. liquid . . . . .9 d

Peach, dried, sulfured:

uncooked:

  2 oz. . . . . 4.6 d

  10 halves, approximately 4.6 oz. . . . . 10.7 d

  halves, ½ cup . . . . 6.6 d

stewed, halves, unsweetened, 1/2 cup . . . . 3.5 d
stewed, halves, sweetened, 1/2 cup . . . . 3.2 d
Peach, frozen:
sliced, sweetened, 5 oz. . . . . 2.0 d
sliced, sweetened, 1/2 cup . . . . 1.8 d
Peach cobbler, see "Cobbler, frozen"
Peach nectar:
canned or bottled, 6 fl. oz. . . . . 1.1 d
Peach pie, see "Pie" and "Pie, snack"
Peanut butter:
chunky, 1 oz. . . . . 1.9 d
chunky, 2 tbsp. . . . . 2.1 d
chunky or creamy (Arrowhead Mills), 2 tbsp. . . . . 4.5 d
chunky or creamy (Peter Pan/Peter Pan Salt
Free), 2 tbsp. . . . . 2.0 d
creamy, 1 oz. . . . . 1.7 d
creamy, 2 tbsp. . . . . 1.9 d
Peanut butter torte, see "Cake"
Peanut flour:
defatted, 1 cup . . . . 2.4 c
Peanut oil:
all varieties 0
Peanuts, all varieties, shelled:
(Beer Nuts), 1 oz. 2.0 d
unroasted, 1 oz. . . . . 2.4 d
unroasted, 1/2 cup . . . . 6.2 d
dry-roasted:
  1 oz. . . . . 2.3 d
  1/2 cup . . . . 5.8 d
  (Flavor House), 1 oz. . . . . 2.0 d
honey-roasted, dry- or oil-roasted (Flavor
House), 1 oz. . . . . 1.0 d
oil-roasted, 1 oz. . . . . 2.6 d
oil-roasted, 1/2 cup . . . . 6.6 d
butter toffee (Flavor House), 1 oz. . . . . <1.0 d

Peanuts *(cont.)*
party, oil-roasted, or Spanish *(Flavor House)*,
  1 oz. . . . . 2.0 d
Pear, fresh:
all varieties, untrimmed, 1 lb. . . . . 10.0 d
with peel, Bartlett, 1 medium, 3½" long,
  approximately 2½ per lb. . . . . 4.0 d
with peel, sliced, ½ cup . . . . 2.0 d
Pear, canned:
in juice, syrup, or water:
  4 oz. . . . . 2.3 d
  ½ cup . . . . 2.5 d
  1 pear half and 1⅔ tbsp. liquid . . . . 1.5 d
  (Hunt's), 4 oz. . . . . <1.0 d
in extra light syrup, diced *(Del Monte Lite)*,
  ½ cup . . . . 1.0 d
in heavy syrup, diced *(Del Monte)*, ½ cup . . . . . . 1.0 d
Pear, dried, sulfured:
uncooked:
  2 oz. . . . . 4.3 d
  10 halves, approximately 6.2 oz. . . . . 13.1 d
  halves, ½ cup . . . . 6.8 d
stewed, halves, unsweetened, ½ cup . . . . 8.2 d
stewed, halves, sweetened, ½ cup . . . . 8.1 d
Pear, Asian:
untrimmed, 1 lb. . . . . 14.9 d
1 medium, 2½" diameter, approximately 4.7 oz.
  untrimmed . . . . 4.4 d
1 large, 3" diameter, approximately 10.7 oz.
  untrimmed . . . . 9.9 d
Pear nectar:
canned or bottled, 6 fl. oz. . . . . 1.1 d
Peas, see specific listings
Peas, cream, canned:
(Allens/East Texas Fair), ½ cup . . . . 3.0 d

Peas, edible-podded, fresh:

raw:

    untrimmed, 1 lb. . . . . 11.1 d

    trimmed, 4 oz. . . . . 3.0 d

    trimmed, ½ cup . . . . 1.9 d

boiled, drained, ½ cup . . . . 2.2 d

Peas, edible-podded, frozen:

unheated, 3.3 oz. . . . . 2.5 d

boiled, drained, ½ cup . . . . 2.4 d

(Green Giant Sugar Snap), ½ cup . . . . 2.0 d

Peas, field, canned:

with snaps *(Allens),* ½ cup . . . . 4.0 d

Peas, green, see "Green peas"

Peas, pepper, see "Pepper peas"

Peas, pigeon, see "Pigeon peas"

Peas, purple hull, see "Purple hull peas"

Peas, snow, Oriental, see "Peas, edible-
    podded"

Peas, split, see "Split peas"

Peas, sprouted, mature seeds:

raw, 4 oz. . . . . 3.2 c

raw, ½ cup . . . . 1.7 c

boiled, drained, 4 oz. 3.7 d

Peas, sweet, see "Green peas"

Peas and carrots, canned:

with liquid, 4 oz. . . . . 3.8 d

with liquid, ½ cup . . . . 4.2 d

Peas and carrots, frozen:

unheated, 3.3 oz. . . . . 3.3 d

unheated, ½ cup . . . . 2.5 d

boiled, drained, ½ cup . . . . 2.4 d

Peas and mushrooms:

(Green Giant Select *Le Sueur),* ½ cup . . . . 4.0 d

Peas and onions, canned:

with liquid, 4 oz. . . . . 1.4 c

with liquid, ½ cup . . . . .7 c

Peas and onions, frozen:

unheated, 3.3 oz. . . . .   3.0 d

unheated, ½ cup . . . .   2.2 d

boiled, drained, ½ cup . . . .   2.7 d

with pearl onions *(Green Giant)*, ½ cup . . . .   4.0 d

Pecans:

dried, in shell, 1 lb. . . . .   18.3 d

dried, shelled:

  1 oz. . . . .   2.2 d

  halves, ½ cup . . . .   4.1 d

  chopped, ½ cup . . . .   4.5 d

  ground, ½ cup . . . .   3.6 d

dry- or oil-roasted, 1 oz. . . . .   .5 c

Pecan cobbler, see "Cobbler, frozen"

Pecan flour:

1 oz. . . . .   .4 c

Pecan pie, see "Pie"

Pectin, dry:

unsweetened, 1.75-oz. package   0

Pepeao, see "Jew's ear"

Pepper, ground:

black, 1 oz. . . . .   7.5 d

black, 1 tsp. . . . .   .6 d

red or cayenne, 1 oz.   7.1 d

red or cayenne, 1 tsp. . . . .   .5 d

seasoned (see also specific listings) *(Lawry's*

  Spice Blends)*, 1 tsp. . . . .   .2 c

Pepper, bell, see "Pepper, sweet"

Pepper, cherry:

plain or pickled *(Progresso)*, ½ cup . . . .   1.0 d

Pepper, chili, green and red, without seeds:

raw, 1 medium, approximately 1.6 oz. . . . .   .7 d

raw, chopped, ½ cup . . . .   1.1 d

Pepper, chili, canned (see also "Jalapeño"):

1 pepper, approximately 2½ oz. . . . .   1.4 d

green, with liquid, chopped, ½ cup . . . .   1.3 d

Pepper, green, see "Pepper, chili," and
  "Pepper, sweet"
Pepper, pepperoncini:
(Progresso Tuscan), ½ cup . . . . 1.0 d
Pepper, piccalilli:
(Progresso), ½ cup . . . . 1.0 d
Pepper, red, see "Pepper, chili," "Pepper,
  sweet," and "Pimiento"
Pepper, sweet, green and red, fresh:
raw:
  untrimmed, 1 lb. 6.7 d
  1 medium, 3″ diameter, approximately 3.2 oz.
    untrimmed . . . . 1.3 d
  chopped, ½ cup .9 d
boiled, drained, 1 medium . . . . .9 d
boiled, drained, chopped, ½ cup . . . . .8 d
Pepper, sweet, in jars (see also "Pimiento"):
with liquid, 4 oz. 1.4 d
with liquid, halves, ½ cup . . . . .8 d
fried *(Progresso),* ½ jar . . . . 1.0 d
roasted *(Progresso),* ½ cup . . . . 1.7 d
Pepper, sweet, freeze-dried, 1 oz. . . . . 4.6 d
Pepper, sweet, frozen:
chopped, 1 oz. . . . . .5 d
Pepper peas, canned:
(Allens/East Texas Fair), ½ cup . . . . 4.0 d
Pepper sauce, hot:
(Gebhardt), ½ tsp. . . . . <1.0 d
(Tabasco), 2 fl. oz. . . . . (0)
cayenne *(Maull's),* 1 tsp. 0
Pepper steak, see "Steak, pepper"
Peppered loaf:
(Kahn's), 1 slice . . . . (0)
(Oscar Mayer), 1 oz. . . . . (0)
Pepperoni:
all varieties, 4 oz. 0

Perch* 0
Persimmon, native:
1 medium, approximately 1.1 oz. . . . . .4 c
Persimmon, Japanese, fresh:
fresh, untrimmed, 1 lb. . . . . 13.7 d
fresh, 1 medium, 2½″ diameter, approximately
  7 oz. untrimmed . . . . 6.0 d
dried, 4 oz. . . . . 16.5 d
dried, 1 medium, approximately 1.3 oz. . . . . 4.9 d
Petite peas, see "Green peas"
Pheasant* 0
Picante beans, canned:
(Allens/East Texas Fair), ½ cup . . . . 5.0 d
Picante sauce (see also "Salsa"):
(Old El Paso Thick'n Chunky), 2 tbsp. . . . . <1.0 d
(Tabasco), 1 oz. . . . . .4 d
hot, medium, or mild *(Rosarita* Chunky), 3 tbsp. . <1.0 d
Pickerel* 0
Pickle, cucumber, in jars:
dill, kosher, Polish, or sour, 4 oz. . . . . 1.4 d
dill, whole, 3¾″ long, approximately 2.3 oz. . . . . . .8 d
dill, 10 slices, approximately 2.1 oz. . . . . .7 d
sour, 1 medium, 3¾″ long, approximately
  1.2 oz. . . . . .4 d
sour, 10 slices, approximately 2.5 oz. . . . . .8 d
sweet:
  4 oz. . . . . 1.3 d
  1 large, 3″ long, approximately 1.2 oz. . . . . .4 d
  10 slices, approximately 2.1 oz. . . . . .7 d
Pickle loaf:
(Kahn's), 1 slice . . . . (0)
Pickle and pimiento loaf:
(Oscar Mayer), 1 slice 0
Pickle relish, see "Relish"
Pickling spice:
(Tone's), 1 tsp. . . . . .3 d

Pie (see also "Pie, snack"):

apple, ⅛ of 9″ pie, approximately 4.4 oz.	2.1 d
cherry, ⅛ of 9″ pie, approximately 4.4 oz.	1.0 d
chocolate cream, ⅙ of 8″ pie, approximately 4 oz.	2.3 d
coconut custard, ⅙ of 8″ pie, approximately 3.7 oz.	1.9 d
egg custard, ⅙ of 8″ pie, approximately 3.7 oz. .	1.3 d
fried, fruit[1], 1 piece, 5″ × 3¾″, approximately 4.5 oz.	3.3 d
lemon meringue, ⅙ of 8″ pie, approximately 4 oz.	1.4 d
pecan, ⅙ of 8″ pie, approximately 4 oz.	4.0 d
pumpkin, ⅙ of 8″ pie, approximately 3.8 oz.	2.9 d

Pie, frozen:

apple:

(Mrs. Smith's, 1 lb. 4 oz.), ⅕ of 8″ pie	2.0 d
(Mrs. Smith's Ready to Serve, 1 lb. 7 oz.), ⅕ of 8″ piee	2.0 d
(Mrs. Smith's, 2 lb. 5 oz.), ⅛ of 9″ pie	2.0 d
or Dutch apple *(Mrs. Smith's, 1 lb. 10 oz.),* ⅙ of 8″ pie	1.0 d
or Dutch apple *(Mrs. Smith's, 2 lb. 14 oz.),* 1/10 of 10″ pie	1.0 d
or Dutch apple crumb *(Mrs. Smith's, 2 lb. 9 oz.), ⅑ of 9″ pie*	2.0 d
apple cranberry *(Mrs. Smith's, 1 lb. 10 oz.),* ⅙ of 8″ pie	1.0 d
blackberry or berry *(Mrs. Smith's, 1 lb. 10 oz.),* ⅙ of 8″ pie	0
blueberry *(Mrs. Smith's, 1 lb. 10 oz.), ⅙ of 8″* pie	1.0 d
blueberry cheese yogurt *(Mrs. Smith's, 1 lb. 1 oz.), ¼ of 7″ pie*	1.0 d

[1] Includes apple, blueberry, cherry, lemon, peach, and strawberry.

Pie, frozen *(cont.)*

Boston cream, 1/6 of 9.5-oz. cake,
  approximately 3.2 oz. . . . . 1.2 d
Boston cream *(Mrs. Smith's),* 1/8 of 8″ pie 0
cherry:
  (Mrs. Smith's, 1 lb. 4 oz.), 1/5 of 8″ pie . . . . . . 1.0 d
  (Mrs. Smith's Ready to Serve, 1 lb. 7 oz.),
    1/5 of 8″ pie . . . . 1.0 d
  (Mrs. Smith's, 1 lb. 10 oz.), 1/6 of 8″ pie . . . . . . 1.0 d
  (Mrs. Smith's, 2 lb. 5 oz.), 1/8 of 9″ pie . . . . . . 1.0 d
  (Mrs. Smith's, 2 lb. 14 oz.), 1/10 of 10″ pie . . . . 1.0 d
coconut custard *(Mrs. Smith's,* 1 lb. 9 oz.),
  1/6 of 8″ pie 0
coconut custard *(Mrs. Smith's,* 2 lb. 12 oz.),
  1/10 of 10″ pie 0
cream, French silk *(Mrs. Smith's,* 1 lb. 8 oz.),
  1/5 of 8″ pie . . . . 1.0 d
lemon meringue *(Mrs. Smith's,* 1 lb. 8 oz.), 1/5 of
  8″ pie 0
mince *(Mrs. Smith's,* 1 lb. 10 oz.), 1/6 of 8″ pie . . . 2.0 d
mince *(Mrs. Smith's,* 2 lb. 14 oz.), 1/10 of 10″ pie . . . 2.0 d
peach *(Mrs. Smith's,* 1 lb. 10 oz.), 1/6 of 8″ pie . . . 1.0 d
peach *(Mrs. Smith's,* 2 lb. 5 oz.), 1/8 of 9″ pie . . . 1.0 d
peach cheese yogurt *(Mrs. Smith's,* 1 lb. 1 oz.),
  1/4 of 7″ pie . . . . 1.0 d
pecan *(Mrs. Smith's,* 1 lb. 8 oz.), 1/5 of 8″ pie . . . 1.0 d
pecan *(Mrs. Smith's,* 2 lb. 4 oz.), 1/10 of 10″ pie . 1.0 d
pumpkin:
  (Mrs. Smith's, 1 lb. 10 oz.), 1/6 of 8″ pie . . . . . . 1.0 d
  (Mrs. Smith's, 2 lb. 14 oz.), 1/10 of 10″ pie . . . . 1.0 d
  hearty *(Mrs. Smith's,* 1 lb. 10 oz.), 1/6 of 8″
    pie . . . . 2.0 d
raspberry, red *(Mrs. Smith's,* 1 lb. 10 oz.), 1/6 of
  8″ pie 0
strawberry *(Mrs. Smith's,* 1 lb. 4 oz.), 1/5 of 8″
  pie . . . . 2.0 d

strawberry banana yogurt *(Mrs. Smith's,*
1 lb. 1 oz.), ¼ of 7" pie . . . .   1.0 d
strawberry rhubarb *(Mrs. Smith's,* 1 lb. 10 oz.),
⅙ of 8" pie   0

Pie, snack:
apple *(Hostess),* 1 piece . . . .   2.0 d
apple *(Tastykake),* 1 piece . . . .   2.0 d
banana or coconut creme *(Tastykake),* 1 piece . . .   2.0 d
blackberry, blueberry, or cherry *(Hostess),*
1 piece . . . .   2.4 d
blueberry or cherry *(Tastykake),* 1 piece . . . .   2.0 d
lemon *(Hostess),* 1 piece . . . .   1.4 d
lemon *(Tastykake),* 1 piece . . . .   2.0 d
lemon-lime or strawberry *(Tastykake),* 1 piece . . .   1.0 d
peach *(Hostess),* 1 piece . . . .   2.0 d
peach *(Tastykake),* 1 piece . . . .   3.0 d
pineapple-cheese or pumpkin *(Tastykake),*
1 piece . . . .   2.0 d
strawberry *(Hostess),* 1 piece . . . .   2.2 d
(Tastykake Tasty Klair), 1 piece . . . .   2.0 d

Pie crust shell:
regular or deep dish *(Stilwell),* ⅛ shell . . . .   1.0 d
graham cracker *(Stilwell),* ⅙ shell . . . .   1.0 d

Pie filling, canned:
apple *(Comstock),* ⅓ cup . . . .   2.0 d
blueberry or cherry *(Comstock),* ⅓ cup . . . .   1.0 d
pumpkin mix, ½ cup . . . .   1.6 c

Pierogi, frozen:
potato cheese *(Golden),* 3 pieces . . . .   2.0 d
potato onion *(Golden),* 3 pieces . . . .   1.0 d

Pigeon peas, fresh:
raw:
in pods, 1 lb. . . . .   9.2 d
shelled, 10 seeds, approximately .14 oz. . . . .   .2 d
shelled, ½ cup . . . .   3.2 d
boiled, drained, ½ cup . . . .   2.2 c

Pigeon peas, mature, dry:

raw, 1 oz. . . . .   4.3 d

raw, 1/2 cup . . . .   15.4 d

boiled, 1/2 cup . . . .   3.9 d

Pig's feet or knuckles:

all varieties, plain or pickled, 4 oz.   0

Pignolia nuts, see "Pine nuts"

Pike*   0

Pili nuts, dried, shelled:

1 oz. . . . .   .8 c

1 cup . . . .   3.4 c

Pimiento, in jars (see also "Pepper, sweet, in jars"):

2 oz. . . . .   .8 c

1 tbsp. . . . .   .1 c

Pimiento spread:

(Price's Light), 1 oz.   0

Piña colada, canned:

6.8-fl.-oz. can . . . .   .2 d

Piña colada mixer:

bottled (Holland House), 4.5 fl. oz. . . . .   (0)

frozen and diluted, with rum (Bacardi), 7 fl. oz.   . . .   (0)

Pine nuts, dried:

pignolias:

   in shell, 1 lb.   15.7 d

   shelled, 1 oz. . . . .   1.3 d

   shelled, 1/2 cup . . . .   3.6 d

   shelled, 1 tbsp.   .5 d

   (Krinos), 1/2 oz.   1.0 d

pinyons:

   in shell, 1 lb. . . . .   27.7 d

   10 kernels . . . .   .1 d

   shelled, 1 oz. . . . .   3.0 d

Pineapple, fresh:

untrimmed, 1 lb. . . . .   2.8 d

trimmed, 1 slice, 3½" diameter × ¾",
   approximately 3 oz. . . . .   1.0 d
trimmed, diced, ½ cup . . . .   .9 d
Pineapple, canned, in juice or syrup:
4 oz. . . . .   .8 d
1 slice and 1¼ tbsp. liquid . . . .   .4 d
chunks, tidbits, or crushed, ½ cup . . . .   .9 d
Pineapple, frozen, sweetened:
5 oz. . . . . 1.6 d
chunks, ½ cup . . . . 1.3 d
Pineapple juice:
canned, bottled, or frozen and diluted, 6 fl. oz. . .   .2 d
frozen concentrate, undiluted, 6 fl. oz. . . . .   .6 d
Pineapple juice drink:
bottled, 6 fl. oz. . . . . (0)
Pineapple-cheese pie, see "Pie, snack"
Pineapple-grapefruit juice drink:
canned or bottled, 6 fl. oz. . . . .   .2 d
Pineapple-orange juice drink:
canned or bottled, 6 fl. oz. . . . .   .2 d
Pink beans, dry:
raw, 1 oz. . . . . 3.6 d
raw, ½ cup . . . . 13.3 d
boiled, ½ cup . . . . 4.5 d
Pinto beans, dry:
uncooked:
   1 oz. . . . . 6.9 d
   ½ cup . . . . 23.4 d
   (Arrowhead Mills), 2 oz. . . . . 11.2 d
boiled, ½ cup . . . . 7.3 d
Pinto beans, canned:
with liquid, 4 oz. . . . . 4.0 d
with liquid, ½ cup . . . . 4.2 d
(Allens/East Texas Fair), ½ cup . . . . 5.0 d
(Eden), ½ cup . . . . 6.4 d

Pinto beans, canned *(cont.)*
(Eden No Salt Added), ½ cup . . . . 6.0 d
(Gebhardt), 4 oz. 5.0 d
(Green Giant/Joan of Arc), ½ cup . . . . 5.0 d
(Hain), 4 oz. . . . . 6.0 d
(Old El Paso), ½ cup . . . . 8.0 d
(Progresso), ½ cup . . . . 6.5 d
Pinto beans, frozen, immature:
unheated, 3.3 oz. 5.4 d
Pinto beans, sprouted:
raw, 4 oz. . . . . 3.1 c
boiled, drained, 4 oz. . . . . 1.1 c
Pinto beans and rice mix:
(Fantastic), prepared, 10 oz. . . . . 8.0 d
Pinyon nuts, see "Pine nuts"
Pistachio nuts:
dried:
   in shell, 1 lb. 24.5 d
   shelled, 1 oz. 3.1 d
   shelled, ½ cup . . . . 6.9 d
dry-roasted:
   in shell, 1 lb. 25.5 d
   shelled, 1 oz. 3.1 d
   shelled, ½ cup . . . . 6.9 d
Pistachio torte, see "Cake"
Pitanga:
1 medium, .3 oz. . . . . <.1 c
½ cup . . . . .5 c
Pizza, frozen:
Canadian bacon *(Totino's Party),* ½ pie . . . . 3.0 d
Canadian bacon *(Jeno's Crisp'N Tasty),*
½ pie . . . . 1.0 d
cheese:
   (Jeno's Crisp'N Tasty), ½ pie . . . . 1.0 d
   (Totino's Party), ½ pie . . . . 2.0 d
   (Totino's Party Family Size), ⅓ pie . . . . 2.0 d

cheese, three:
   (Pappalo's, 9"), ¹/₂ pie . . . . 4.0 d
   (Pappalo's, 12"), ¹/₄ pie . . . . 4.0 d
   (Pappalo's Pan), ¹/₅ pie . . . . 3.0 d
combination:
   (Jeno's Crisp'N Tasty), ¹/₂ pie . . . . 1.0 d
   (Totino's Party), ¹/₂ pie . . . . 3.0 d
   (Totino's Party Family Size), ¹/₃ pie . . . . 3.0 d
hamburger *(Jeno's Crisp'N Tasty),* ¹/₂ pie . . . . . . 1.0 d
hamburger *(Totino's Party),* ¹/₂ pie . . . . 3.0 d
pepperoni:
   (Jeno's Crisp'N Tasty), ¹/₂ pie . . . . 1.0 d
   (Pappalo's, 9"), ¹/₂ pie . . . . 4.0 d
   (Pappalo's, 12"), ¹/₄ pie . . . . 4.0 d
   (Pappalo's Pan), ¹/₅ pie . . . . 3.0 d
   (Tombstone Light), ¹/₂ pie . . . . 2.0 d
   (Totino's Party), ¹/₂ pie . . . . 3.0 d
   (Totino's Party Family Size), ¹/₃ pie . . . . 3.0 d
sausage:
   (Jeno's Crisp'N Tasty), ¹/₂ pie . . . . 1.0 d
   (Pappalo's, 9"), ¹/₂ pie . . . . 4.0 d
   (Pappalo's, 12"), ¹/₄ pie . . . . 4.0 d
   (Pappalo's Pan), ¹/₅ pie . . . . 3.0 d
   (Totino's Party), ¹/₂ pie . . . . 3.0 d
   (Totino's Party Family Size), ¹/₃ pie . . . . 4.0 d
sausage and pepperoni:
   (Pappalo's, 9"), ¹/₂ pie . . . . 4.0 d
   (Pappalo's, 12"), ¹/₄ pie . . . . 4.0 d
   (Pappalo's Pan), ¹/₅ pie . . . . 3.0 d
supreme:
   (Pappalo's, 9"), ¹/₂ pie . . . . 4.0 d
   (Pappalo's, 12"), ¹/₄ pie . . . . 4.0 d
   (Pappalo's Pan), ¹/₅ pie . . . . 3.0 d
   (Tombstone Light), ¹/₂ pie . . . . 2.0 d
   (Tombstone Light, 12"), ¹/₅ pie . . . . 4.0 d

Pizza *(cont.)*

vegetable *(Tombstone* Light), ½ pie . . . .   2.0 d
vegetable *(Tombstone* Light), 12″), ⅕ pie . . . . . .   3.0 d

Pizza Hut:

hand-tossed, 1 slice (⅛ pie):

   beef or pork . . . .   2.7 d
   cheese . . . .   2.5 d
   Meat Lover's or Pepperoni Lover's . . . .   2.7 d
   pepperoni . . . .   2.2 d
   sausage, Italian . . . .   2.5 d
   supreme . . . .   3.2 d
   super supreme . . . .   2.8 d
   Veggie Lover's . . . .   2.9 d

pan pizza, 1 slice (⅛ pie):

   beef or pork . . . .   2.7 d
   cheese . . . .   2.5 d
   Meat Lover's or Pepperoni Lover's . . . .   2.7 d
   pepperoni . . . .   2.2 d
   sausage, Italian . . . .   2.5 d
   supreme . . . .   3.2 d
   super supreme . . . .   2.8 d
   Veggie Lover's . . . .   2.9 d

Thin 'n Crispy, 1 slice (⅛ pie):

   beef or pork . . . .   2.3 d
   cheese . . . .   2.1 d
   Meat Lover's or Pepperoni Lover's . . . .   2.3 d
   pepperoni . . . .   1.8 d
   sausage, Italian . . . .   2.1 d
   supreme . . . .   2.8 d
   super supreme or Veggie Lover's . . . .   2.5 d

Pizza roll, frozen:

cheese, *(Jeno's Pizza Rolls),* 3 oz. . . . .   1.4 d
combination, *(Jeno's Pizza Rolls),* 3 oz. . . . .   1.9 d
hamburger, *(Jeno's Pizza Rolls),* 3 oz. . . . .   2.0 d
pepperoni, *(Jeno's Pizza Rolls),* 3 oz. . . . .   1.8 d
sausage, *(Jeno's Pizza Rolls),* 3 oz. . . . .   1.6 d

Pizza sauce:
(Pastorelli Continental Chef), ¼ cup . . . .   3.0 d
(Pastorelli Italian Chef), 2 oz. . . . .   2.0 d
Plantain, fresh:
raw:
    untrimmed, 1 lb.   6.8 d
    1 medium, approximately 9.7 oz. untrimmed   .   4.1 d
    sliced, ½ cup . . . .   1.7 d
cooked, sliced, ½ cup . . . .   1.8 d
Plum, fresh, with peel:
untrimmed, 1 lb. . . . .   2.7 d
Japanese or hybrid, 1 medium, 2⅛" diameter,
    approximately 2.5 oz. . . . .   1.0 d
pitted, sliced, ½ cup . . . .   1.2 d
Plum, canned:
in juice, syrup, or water, 4 oz. . . . .   1.1 d
in juice, syrup, or water, ½ cup . . . .   1.3 d
in juice or water, 3 plums and 2 tbsp. liquid . . . .   1.0 d
in light or heavy syrup, 3 plums and 2¾ tbsp.
    liquid . . . .   1.3 d
Poi:
½ cup . . . .   .5 d
Poke greens, canned:
(Allens), ½ cup . . . .   1.0 d
Pokeberry shoots:
raw, 4 oz. . . . .   1.9 d
raw, ½ cup . . . .   1.4 d
boiled, drained, ½ cup . . . .   1.2 d
Polenta mix:
(Fantastic), 4 oz. . . . .   .3 d
Polish sausage:
all varieties   0
Pollock*   0
Pomegranate:
untrimmed, 1 lb. . . . .   1.5 d

Pomegranate *(cont.)*
1 medium, 3⅜″ diameter, approximately 9.7 oz.
untrimmed . . . . .9 d
Pompano* 0
Popcorn, popped:
(Jiffy Pop Pan Popcorn), 4 cups . . . . 2.0 d
(Kettle Poppins), ½ oz. . . . . 1.0 d
(Orville Redenbacher's Gourmet Hot Air),
3 cups . . . . 3.0 d
(Orville Redenbacher's Gourmet Original/White),
3 cups . . . . 3.0 d
butter *(Cape Cod),* ½ oz. . . . . 1.0 d
butter flavor *(Jiffy Pop* Pan Popcorn), 4 cups . . . 2.0 d
caramel crunch *(Flavor House),* 1.1 oz. . . . . 1.0 d
cheddar, white *(Flavor House),* 1.1 oz. . . . . 2.0 d
air popped, white or yellow *(Jolly Time),* 3 cups . 4.0 d
Popcorn, microwave, popped:
plain or butter flavor *(Jiffy Pop* Pan), 4 cups . . . . 2.0 d
(Jolly Time Natural/Natural Light), 3 cups . . . . . . 3.0 d
(Orville Redenbacher's Gourmet Natural/Salt
Free/Light), 3 cups . . . . 3.0 d
(Pop · Secret/Pop · Secret Light), 3 cups . . . . . . 2.0 d
(Pop Weaver's Natural/Butter), 4 cups . . . . 4.0 d
butter flavor:
(Jolly Time/Jolly Time Light), 3 cups . . . . 3.0 d
(Orville Redenbacher's Gourmet/Salt Free/
Lite), 3 cups . . . . 3.0 d
(Pop · Secret/Pop · Secret Light/Salt Free),
3 cups . . . . 2.0 d
butter toffee or caramel *(Orville Redenbacher's*
Gourmet), 2½ cups . . . . 2.0 d
cheddar or sour cream 'n onion *(Orville
Redenbacher's* Gourmet), 3 cups . . . . 3.0 d
Popcorn seasoning:
(Tone's), 1 tsp. 0

Poppy seeds:

1 oz. . . . . 8.3 d

1 tsp. . . . . .8 d

Porgy* 0

Pork* 0

Pork, sweet and sour, canned:

(La Choy), ³⁄₄ cup . . . . 1.0 d

Pork chow mein, canned:

(La Choy Bi-Pack), ³⁄₄ cup . . . . 2.0 d

Pork gravy, canned:

(Heinz Home Style), ¹⁄₄ cup . . . . .1 d

Pork and beans, see "Baked beans"

Pot roast seasoning mix:

(Lawry's Seasoning Blends), 1 package . . . . .5 c

Pork sausage:

all varieties, 4 oz. 0

Potato:

raw:

  untrimmed, 1 lb. . . . . 5.4 d

  peeled, 2¹⁄₂"-diameter potato . . . . 1.8 d

  peeled, diced, ¹⁄₂ cup . . . . 1.2 d

baked:

  in skin, 1 medium, 4³⁄₄" × 2¹⁄₃" diameter,

    approximately 7 oz. . . . . 4.8 d

  baked, pulp only, 4 oz. . . . . 1.7 d

  baked, pulp only, ¹⁄₂ cup . . . . .9 d

  skin only, from 4³⁄₄"-long potato,

    approximately 2 oz. . . . . 2.3 d

boiled in skin, peeled:

  2¹⁄₂"-diameter potato, approximately 5.3 oz. . . . 2.4 d

  4 oz. . . . . 2.0 d

  ¹⁄₂ cup . . . . 1.4 d

boiled without skin, 2¹⁄₂"-diameter potato . . . . . . 2.4 d

microwaved in skin:

  1 medium, 4³⁄₄" × 2¹⁄₃" diameter . . . . 1.6 c

  4 oz. . . . . .9 c

Potato, microwaved in skin *(cont.)*

peeled, ½ cup . . . . .3 c

skin only, 2 oz. . . . . 1.8 c

hash brown, ½ cup . . . . 1.6 d

mashed, with milk and butter or margarine,

½ cup . . . . 2.1 d

Potato, canned:

with liquid, 4 oz. . . . . 1.8 d

with liquid, ½ cup . . . . 2.4 d

whole, new *(Hunt's)*, 4 oz. . . . . <1.0 d

Potato, frozen:

whole, unheated, ½ cup or 3.3 oz., ⅓ of 10-oz.

package . . . . 2.6 d

french fried, par-fried:

unheated, 3 oz., ⅓ of 9-oz. package . . . . 2.0 d

heated, 10 strips, approximately 2.3 oz. . . . . . . .5 d

crinkle cut *(MicroMagic)*, 3 oz. . . . . 1.0 d

sticks *(MicroMagic Tater Sticks)*, 4 oz. . . . . . . 1.0 d

hash brown:

unheated, 4 oz. . . . . 1.6 d

unheated, ½ cup . . . . 1.5 d

heated, ½ cup . . . . 1.6 d

(MicroMagic Okray), 3 oz. . . . . 1.0 d

mashed *(Simplot Singles)*, 4 oz. . . . . 1.0 d

O'Brien, unheated, 4 oz. . . . . 2.2 d

pancake, see "Potato pancake"

puffs:

unheated, 4 oz. . . . . 2.6 d

prepared, 10 puffs, approximately 2.5 oz. . . . . 2.2 d

prepared, ½ cup . . . . 2.0 d

and broccoli, with cheese sauce *(Green Giant*

One Serving), 5.5 oz. . . . . 2.0 d

Potato, mix, prepared, except as noted:

au gratin:

dry, 5½-oz. package . . . . 10.3 d

(Fantastic Foods), ½ cup . . . .   1.7 d
tangy *(Pillsbury)*, ½ cup . . . .   1.0 d
cheddar and bacon *(Pillsbury)*, ½ cup . . . .   1.0 d
country style *(Fantastic Foods)*, ½ cup . . . .   1.7 d
mashed:
  flakes, dry, ½ cup . . . .   1.5 d
  (Hungry Jack Flakes), ½ cup . . . .   1.0 d
  (Pillsbury Idaho Granules/*Pillsbury Idaho*
    Spuds), ½ cup . . . .   1.0 d
pancake, see "Potato pancake"
scalloped, dry, 5½-oz. package . . . .   13.4 d
scalloped, cheesy or creamy white sauce
  (Pillsbury), ½ cup . . . .   1.0 d
sour cream and chives *(Pillsbury)*, ½ cup . . . . .   1.0 d
Potato, sweet, see "Sweet potato"
Potato chips:
all varieties *(Lay's)*, 1 oz. . . . .   1.1 d
all varieties *(Ruffles)*, 1 oz. . . . .   1.1 d
Potato flour:
1 cup . . . .   10.9 d
Potato pancake:
frozen *(Golden)*, 1 cake . . . .   1.0 d
mix, prepared *(Pillsbury)*, 3 cakes, 3″ each . . . . .   1.0 d
Potato salad seasoning:
(Tone's), 1 tsp. . . . .   .1 d
Potato sticks:
1 oz. . . . .   .3 c
Potatoes au gratin:
packaged *(Green Giant Pantry Express)*, ½ cup .   1.5 d
mix, see "Potato, mix"
Potherb, see "Jute"
Poultry*   0
Poultry seasoning:
1 oz. . . . .   3.2 d
1 tsp. . . . .   .2 d

Pout, ocean* 0
Preserves, see "Jam and preserves"
Pretzels (see also "Crackers"):
hard, plain, 1 oz. . . . . .8 d
whole wheat, hard, 1 oz. . . . . .5 c
Pretzels, frozen:
(Super-Pretzel), 1 piece . . . . 3.0 d
Prickly pear:
untrimmed, 1 lb. . . . . 12.3 d
1 medium, approximately 4.8 oz. untrimmed . . . . 3.7 d
Prosciutto:
all varieties, 4 oz. 0
Prune, canned, in heavy syrup:
pitted, 4 oz. . . . . 4.3 d
½ cup . . . . 4.4 d
5 medium and 2 tbsp. syrup . . . . 3.3 d
Prune, dehydrated:
uncooked, ½ cup . . . . 1.9 c
cooked, ½ cup . . . . 1.4 c
Prune, dried:
uncooked:
  with pits, 2 oz. . . . . 3.5 d
  with pits, ½ cup . . . . 5.7 d
  pitted, 2 oz. . . . . 4.0 d
  pitted, 10 prunes . . . . 6.0 d
stewed, with pits, unsweetened, ½ cup . . . . 7.0 d
stewed, with pits, sweetened, ½ cup . . . . 4.5 d
Prune juice:
canned or bottled, 6 fl. oz. . . . . 1.9 d
Pudding, ready-to-serve:
all varieties:
  (Hunt's Snack Pack Light), 4 oz. 0
  (Swiss Miss/Swiss Miss Light), 4 oz. 0
  except lemon *(Hunt's Snack Pack),* 4.25 oz. 0
lemon *(Hunt's Snack Pack),* 4.25 oz. . . . . <1.0 d

Pudding, frozen:
butterscotch or vanilla *(Rich's)*, 3 oz. 0
chocolate *(Rich's)*, 3 oz. . . . . .2 d
Pudding mix, prepared:
chocolate, ½ cup . . . . 1.5 d
Pummelo:
untrimmed, 1 lb. . . . . 2.5 d
1 medium, 5½" diameter, approximately
   2.4 lbs. untrimmed . . . . 6.1 d
trimmed, sections, ½ cup . . . . 1.0 d
Pumpkin, fresh:
raw, untrimmed, 1 lb. 5.7 d
raw, pulp, 1" cubes, ½ cup . . . . 1.0 d
boiled, drained, mashed, ½ cup . . . . 1.0 d
Pumpkin, canned:
(Libby's), ½ cup . . . . 3.8 d
with or without winter squash, 4 oz. . . . . 3.2 d
with or without winter squash, ½ cup . . . . 3.4 d
for pie, see "Pie filling"
Pumpkin flower:
raw, untrimmed, 1 lb. 1.0 c
raw, ½ cup . . . . .1 c
boiled, drained, ½ cup . . . . .6 d
Pumpkin leaf:
raw, untrimmed, 1 lb. 1.9 c
raw, ½ cup . . . . .2 c
boiled, drained, ½ cup . . . . .9 d
Pumpkin pie, see "Pie"
Pumpkin pie spice:
1 oz. . . . . 4.2 d
1 tsp. . . . . .3 d
Pumpkin seed kernels:
roasted, 1 oz. . . . . 1.8 d
roasted, ½ cup . . . . 7.4 d
dried, 1 oz. . . . . 3.9 d
dried, ½ cup . . . . 9.5 d

Punch, see "Fruit punch"

Purple hull peas, canned:

(Allens/East Texas Fair), ½ cup . . . .   4.0 d

Purslane:

raw, untrimmed, 1 lb. . . . .   2.7 c

raw, ½ cup . . . .   .2 c

boiled, drained, ½ cup . . . .   .5 c

Q

Food and Measure	Fiber Grams

Quail* 0
Quince:
untrimmed, 1 lb. . . . . 5.3 d
1 medium, approximately 5.3 oz. untrimmed . . . . 1.7 d
peeled and seeded, 1 oz. . . . . .5 d
Quinoa, dry:
2 oz. . . . . 3.3 d
½ cup . . . . 5.0 d
(Eden), 2 oz. . . . . 4.3 d

R

Food and Measure	Fiber Grams
Rabbit*	0
Radish, raw:	
untrimmed, 1 lb.	6.5 d
10 medium, ¾″ to 1″ diameter, approximately	
1.6 oz. untrimmed	.7 d
sliced, ½ cup	.9 d
Radish, Oriental:	
raw:	
untrimmed, 1 lb.	5.7 d
1 medium, 7″ × 2¼″ diameter, approximately	
15 oz. untrimmed	5.4 d
trimmed, sliced, ½ cup	.7 d
boiled, drained, sliced, ½ cup	1.2 d
Radish, Oriental, dried:	
1 oz.	2.4 c
Radish, white-icicle, raw:	
1 medium, .6 oz.	.1 c
sliced, ½ cup	.4 c
Raisins, regular or golden:	
seeded:	
2 oz.	3.9 d
½ cup not packed	4.9 d
½ cup packed	5.6 d
seedless:	
2 oz.	2.3 d

½ cup not packed . . . .   2.9 d
½ cup packed . . . .   3.3 d
Raspberry juice drink, blend:
bottled, 6 fl. oz. . . . .   (0)
Raspberry-tamarind sauce:
dipping *(Helen's Tropical Exotics)*, 2 tbsp. . . . . . .   1.0 d
Raspberry pie, see "Pie"
Raspberries, red, fresh:
1 pint . . . .   21.2 d
4 oz. . . . .   7.8 d
½ cup . . . .   4.2 d
Raspberries, canned:
in heavy syrup, 4 oz. . . . .   3.8 d
in heavy syrup, ½ cup . . . .   4.2 d
Raspberries, frozen:
sweetened, 5 oz.   6.2 d
sweetened, ½ cup . . . .   5.5 d
in syrup *(Birds Eye)*, 5 oz. . . . .   4.0 d
Ravioli, frozen:
mini *(Celentano)*, 4 oz. . . . .   2.0 d
Red bean mix:
and rice, prepared *(Fantastic* Cajun), 10 oz. . . . .   9.0 d
Red beans (see also "Kidney beans"), canned:
(Allens), ½ cup . . . .   5.0 d
(Green Giant/Joan of Arc), ½ cup . . . .   5.0 d
small *(Hunt's)*, 4 oz. . . . .   6.0 d
Red snapper*   0
Redfish*   0
Refried beans, canned:
4 oz. . . . .   6.0 d
½ cup . . . .   6.7 d
(Gebhardt), 4 oz.   6.8 d
(Old El Paso), 4 oz. . . . .   5.0 d
with bacon, nacho cheese, chilies, or onions
    (Rosarita), 4 oz.   6.0 d
with green chilies *(Old El Paso)*, ¼ cup . . . .   2.5 d

Refried beans, canned *(cont.)*

with green chilies, jalapeño *(Gebhardt)*, 4 oz.	6.8 d
plain (vegetarian), or spicy *(Rosarita)*, 4 oz.	6.0 d
vegetarian *(Hain)*, 4 oz.	5.0 d
vegetarian *(Old El Paso)*, 4 oz.	5.0 d

Refried bean mix:

(Fantastic Instant), prepared, ½ cup	12.0 d

Relish, pickle:

hamburger:

1 oz.	.9 d
¼ cup	2.0 d
1 tbsp.	.5 d
hot dog, ¼ cup	.5 c
jalapeño *(Old El Paso)*, 2 tbsp.	1.0 d
sweet, ¼ cup	.5 c

Rhubarb, fresh:

raw, untrimmed, 1 lb.	6.1 d
trimmed, diced, ½ cup	1.1 d

Rhubarb, frozen:

uncooked, 5 oz.	2.6 d
cooked, sweetened, ½ cup	2.4 d

Rice:

basmati, see "Rice, basmati"

brown, long grain, uncooked:

2 oz.	2.0 d
½ cup	3.2 d
(Arrowhead Mills), 2 oz.	3.1 d
(Uncle Ben's Whole Grain), 1.3 oz.	1.0 d
(Uncle Ben's Fast Cooking Whole Grain), .9 oz.	.8 d
brown, long grain, cooked, ½ cup	1.8 d
brown, medium or short grain *(Arrowhead Mills)*, 2 oz. dry	3.4 d

jasmine, see "Rice, jasmine"

glutinous or sweet:

uncooked, 2 oz.	1.6 d

uncooked, ½ cup	2.6 d
cooked, ½ cup	1.2 d
white, long grain, regular:	
uncooked, 2 oz.	.7 d
uncooked, ½ cup	1.2 d
cooked, ½ cup	.1 c
white, long grain, parboiled:	
uncooked, 2 oz.	1.0 d
uncooked, ½ cup	1.6 d
uncooked (*Uncle Ben's Converted*),	
1.2 oz. dry	.3 d
cooked, ½ cup	.4 d
white, long grain, precooked or instant:	
uncooked, 2 oz.	.9 d
uncooked, ½ cup	.8 d
uncooked (*Uncle Ben's* Boil-In-Bag), 1 oz.	.5 d
uncooked (*Uncle Ben's* Fast Cooking),	
1.1 oz. dry	.4 d
cooked, ½ cup	.5 d
white, medium grain:	
uncooked, 2 oz.	.8 d
uncooked, ½ cup	1.4 d
cooked, ½ cup	.3 d
white, short grain, uncooked, 2 oz.	1.6 d
white, short grain, uncooked, ½ cup	2.8 d
wild, see "Wild rice"	
Rice, basmati:	
brown:	
uncooked (*Arrowhead Mills*), 2 oz.	3.1 d
cooked (*Fantastic Foods*), ½ cup	.4 d
cooked (*Master Choice Texmati*), ½ cup	1.0 d
white, cooked (*Fantastic Foods*), ½ cup	.3 d
white, cooked (*Master Choice Texmati*), ½ cup	.2 d
white and wild, cooked (*Master Choice*	
Texmati), ½ cup	1.0 d

Rice, fried, canned:

(La Choy), ¾ cup . . . . <1.0 d

Rice, jasmine, cooked:

(Fantastic Foods), ½ cup . . . . .3 d

brown *(Fantastic Foods),* ½ cup . . . . .4 d

Rice, wild, see "Wild rice"

Rice bran, crude:

1 oz. . . . . 6.0 d

½ cup . . . . 8.7 d

1 tbsp. . . . . 1.1 d

Rice and broccoli, frozen:

in cheese sauce *(Green Giant* One Serving),

   5.5 oz. . . . . 2.0 d

Rice cake:

brown rice, plain, 1 oz. . . . . 1.2 d

brown rice, sesame, 1 oz. . . . . 1.5 d

Rice dishes, mix, unprepared, except as noted:

au gratin, herbed *(Country Inn),* 1.2 oz. . . . . .7 d

broccoli:

  almondine *(Country Inn),* 1.2 oz. . . . . .8 d

  au gratin *(Country Inn),* 1.1 oz. . . . . .9 d

  and cheddar, white *(Country Inn),* 1.2 oz. . . . . . .8 d

brown:

  plain or Spanish *(Arrowhead Mills* Quick

    Brown Rice), 2 oz. . . . . 2.8 d

  vegetable herb *(Arrowhead Mills* Quick

    Brown Rice), 2 oz. . . . . 4.0 d

  and wild, herb *(Arrowhead Mills* Quick Brown

    Rice), 2 oz. . . . . 4.0 d

chicken flavor:

  creamy, and mushroom *(Country Inn),* 1.3 oz. . 1.0 d

  creamy, and wild rice *(Country Inn),* 1.3 oz. . . . . .6 d

  stock *(Country Inn),* 1.2 oz. . . . . .5 d

  and vegetables, homestyle *(Country Inn),*

    1.3 oz. . . . . .9 d

Florentine *(Country Inn),* 1.2 oz. . . . . .9 d

green bean almondine *(Country Inn)*, 1.2 oz. . . . . . .8 d
long grain and wild:
   (Uncle Ben's Original), 1 oz. . . . . .6 d
   (Uncle Ben's Original Fast Cook), 1 oz. . . . . . . .8 d
   chicken stock sauce *(Uncle Ben's)*, 1.3 oz. . . . 1.1 d
with pasta, seasoned, ½ cup prepared . . . . . . 3.9 d
pilaf, brown, with miso or Spanish *(Quick Pilaf)*,
   ½ cup prepared . . . . .5 d
pilaf, vegetable *(Country Inn)*, 1.2 oz. . . . . .7 d
Spanish, and beans *(Fantastic Only a Pinch)*,
   10 oz. prepared . . . . 8.0 d
vegetable blend, garden *(Uncle Ben's)*, 1.3 oz. . . . . .9 d
Rice flour:
brown:
   2 oz. . . . . 2.6 d
   ½ cup . . . . 3.6 d
   (Arrowhead Mills), 2 oz. . . . . 3.1 d
white, 2 oz. . . . . 1.4 d
white, ½ cup . . . . 1.9 d
Rockfish* 0
Roe* 0
Rolls (see also "Rolls, sweet"):
(Arnold Bakery Light), 1 piece . . . . 4.0 d
(Arnold Bran'nola Buns), 1 piece . . . . 3.0 d
(Wonder Enriched Buns), 1 piece . . . . .7 d
brown and serve:
   (Pepperidge Farm Hearth), 1 piece 0
   (Roman Meal), 1 piece . . . . 1.2 d
   Bavarian wheat *(Bread du Jour)*, 1 piece . . . . 1.6 d
   plain or buttermilk *(Wonder)*, 1 piece . . . . .6 d
   club *(Pepperidge Farm)*, 1 piece 0
   dinner type, 1-oz. piece . . . . .9 d
   Italian, crusty *(Bread du Jour)*, 1 piece . . . . . . .8 d
crescent, butter *(Pepperidge Farm* Heat &
   Serve), 1 piece 0
croissant, see "Croissant"

Rolls *(cont.)*
dinner:

(Pepperidge Farm Country Style/Party),
   1 piece 0

(Roman Meal), 1 piece . . . . 1.2 d

(Wonder), 1 piece .6 d

   parker house, poppy or sesame seed finger
      (Pepperidge Farm), 1 piece 0

   plain or sesame *(Arnold)*, 1 piece . . . . 1.0 d

   potato *(Pepperidge Farm* Hearty), 1 piece . . . . 1.0 d

   (Home Pride), 1 piece . . . . .7 d

egg, dinner type, 2½" piece, approximately
   1.2 oz. . . . . 1.3 d

egg, Dutch *(Arnold)*, 1 piece . . . . 2.0 d

French style, plain or sourdough *(Pepperidge
   Farm)*, 1 piece 0

French style, 7 grain *(Pepperidge Farm)*,
   1 piece . . . . 1.0 d

hamburger:

   (Arnold), 1 piece . . . . 2.0 d

   (Pepperidge Farm), 1 piece 0

   (Roman Meal), 1 piece . . . . 1.9 d

   (Wonder Light), 1 piece . . . . 4.6 d

hamburger or hot dog, mixed grain,
   1½-oz. piece . . . . 1.8 d

hamburger or hot dog, reduced calorie,
   1½-oz. piece . . . . 2.7 d

hoagie, soft *(Pepperidge Farm)*, 1 piece . . . . . . 1.0 d

honey wheat *(Wonder* Buns), 1 piece . . . . 2.1 d

hot dog:

   (Arnold, 12 oz.), 1 piece . . . . 1.0 d

   (Arnold Bran'nola/New England), 1 piece . . . . . 1.0 d

   (Pepperidge Farm), 1 piece 0

   (Roman Meal), 1 piece . . . . 1.8 d

   (Wonder Light), 1 piece . . . . 4.6 d

Dijon *(Pepperidge Farm)*, 1 piece . . . .   2.0 d
sliced *(Brownberry)*, 1 piece . . . .   1.0 d
Italian *(Savoni 8″)*, 1 piece . . . .   3.0 d
kaiser *(August Bros.)*, 1 piece . . . .   2.0 d
kaiser *(Brownberry* Hearth), 1 piece . . . .   2.0 d
oat bran, dinner type, 1½-oz. piece . . . .   1.7 d
onion *(Arnold* Premium/Soft), 1 piece . . . .   2.0 d
onion *(August Bros.)*, 1 piece . . . .   2.0 d
pan *(Wonder)*, 1 piece . . . .   .6 d
pan Cubano *(Arnold Agusto)*, 1 piece . . . .   2.0 d
party, petite *(Arnold)*, 2 pieces . . . .   1.0 d
potato *(Arnold)*, 1 piece . . . .   2.0 d
sandwich:
  (Roman Meal), 1 piece . . . .   3.4 d
  onion with poppy seeds *(Pepperidge Farm)*,
    1 piece   0
  plain or sesame *(Arnold)*, 1 piece . . . .   2.0 d
  potato *(Pepperidge Farm)*, 1 piece . . . .   1.0 d
  with sesame seeds *(Pepperidge Farm)*,
    1 piece   0
  wheat or white *(Brownberry)*, 1 piece . . . .   2.0 d
sesame *(August Bros.)*, 1 piece . . . .   2.0 d
twist, golden *(Pepperidge Farm* Heat & Serve),
  1 piece   0
Rolls, sweet (see also "Buns, sweet"):
apple cinnamon *(Aunt Fanny's* Old Fashioned),
  1 piece . . . .   1.5 d
caramel nut *(Aunt Fanny's)*, 1 piece . . . .   1.0 d
cinnamon:
  (Aunt Fanny's), 2-oz. piece . . . .   1.0 d
  (Aunt Fanny's Duos), 1 piece . . . .   1.0 d
  (Awrey's Homestyle), 1 piece . . . .   1.0 d
  with raisins, 1 medium, 2¾″ square,
    approximately 2.1 oz. . . . .   .8 d
  swirl *(Awrey's* Grande), 1 piece . . . .   1.0 d

Rolls, sweet (cont.)
fruit roll (Aunt Fanny's Dixie), 1 piece . . . .   1.0 d
pecan twirl (Aunt Fanny's), 1 piece . . . .   1.0 d
Rosé wine:
all varieties, regular or sparkling   0
Roseapple:
trimmed, 1 oz. . . . .   .3 c
Roselle:
1 oz. or ½ cup . . . .   .3 c
Rosemary, dried:
1 tsp. . . . .   .2 c
Rotini entree, frozen:
cheddar (Green Giant Garden Gourmet Right
for Lunch), 9.5 oz.   4.5 d
Roughy, orange*   0
Rutabaga:
raw, untrimmed, 1 lb. . . . .   9.6 d
raw, cubed, ½ cup . . . .   1.8 d
boiled, drained, cubed, ½ cup . . . .   1.5 d
boiled, drained, mashed, ½ cup . . . .   2.2 d
Rye, whole grain:
2 oz. . . . .   8.3 d
½ cup . . . .   12.3 d
(Arrowhead Mills), 2 oz. . . . .   7.6 d
Rye flakes:
(Arrowhead Mills), 2 oz. . . . .   7.6 d
Rye flour:
dark, 2 oz. . . . .   12.8 d
dark, ½ cup . . . .   14.5 d
medium or light, 2 oz. . . . .   8.3 d
medium or light, 1 cup . . . .   7.4 d
medium (Pillsbury's Best), 1 cup . . . .   9.0 d
Rye whiskey:
all varieties   0

S

Food and Measure	Fiber Grams

Sablefish* 0
Safflower oil:
all varieties 0
Safflower seed kernels:
dried, 1 oz. . . . . .7 c
Safflower seed meal:
partially defatted, 1 oz. . . . . 2.2 c
Saffron:
1 oz. . . . . 1.1 d
1 tsp. . . . . <.1 d
Sage, ground:
1 oz. . . . . 5.1 d
1 tsp. . . . . .1 d
Salad dressing:
blue cheese *(La Martinique),* 2 tbsp. 0
Caesar *(Lawry's* Classic), 1 oz. . . . . .1 c
Chinese vinaigrette *(Lawry's* Classic), 1 oz. 0
Dijon, golden *(Lawry's* Classic), 1 oz. 0
French, low calorie, 2 tbsp. . . . . .1 d
Italian *(Ott's),* 1.1 oz. 0
Italian, with Parmesan or blue cheese *(Lawrey's*
   Classic), 1 oz. . . . . .1 c
mayonnaise type, 2 tbsp. 0
oil and vinegar, 2 tbsp. 0

Salad dressing (cont.)

(Ott's Famous), 1.1 oz. 0

poppyseed (La Martinique Original), 2 tbsp. 0

poppyseed or ranch (Ott's), 1.1 oz. 0

red or rice wine vinaigrette (Lawry's Classic),
1 oz. 0

Russian, low calorie, 2 tbsp. . . . . .1 d

San Francisco, with Romano (Lawry's Classic),
1 oz. . . . . .1 c

sesame seed, 1 tbsp. . . . . .1 c

Thousand Island, 2 tbsp. .4 d

vinaigrette, 1 tbsp. 0

vintage, with sherry wine (Lawry's Classic),
1 oz. . . . . .1 c

white wine vinaigrette (Lawry's Classic), 1 oz. . . . . . .1 c

Salami:

all varieties, 4 oz. 0

Salmon* 0

Salmon oil:

all varieties 0

Salsa (see also "Picante sauce" and "Taco
sauce"):

green chili (Old El Paso Thick'n Chunky),
2 tbsp. 0

hot, medium, or mild (Rosarita), 3 tbsp. . . . . <1.0 d

taco, medium, or mild (Rosarita), 3 tbsp. . . . . . . <1.0 d

Texas (Hot Cha Cha), 1 oz. . . . . .4 d

verde (Old El Paso Thick'n Chunky), 2 tbsp. . . . . 1.0 d

Salsa seasoning mix:

(Lawry's Seasoning Blends), 1 package . . . . 1.1 d

Salsify:

raw, untrimmed, 1 lb. . . . . 13.0 d

raw, trimmed, sliced, ½ cup . . . . 2.2 d

boiled, drained, sliced, ½ cup . . . . 2.1 d

Salt:

plain, iodized, or sea, 1 tbsp. 0

Salt, seasoned (see also specific listings):
(Lawry's/Lawry's Light/Spice Blends), 1 tsp. . . . . . .1 c
Salt, substitute or imitation:
(Lawry's Salt-Free 17), 1 tsp. . . . . .4 c
seasoned *(Lawry's Salt-Free)*, 1 tsp. . . . . <.1 c
Salt pork* 0
Sandwich sauce (see also specific listings):
(Hunt's Manwich Extra Thick & Chunky), 2.5 oz. . 2.0 d
(Hunt's Manwich Extra Thick & Chunky),
   prepared, 1 sandwich . . . . 3.0 d
Mexican *(Hunt's Manwich)*, 2.5 oz. . . . . 1.0 d
Mexican *(Hunt's Manwich)*, prepared,
   1 sandwich . . . . 2.0 d
Sloppy Joe *(Hunt's Manwich)*, 2.5 oz. . . . . 1.0 d
Sloppy Joe *(Hunt's Manwich)*, prepared,
   1 sandwich . . . . 1.0 d
Sandwich seasoning mix:
dry *(Hunt's Manwich)*, .25 oz. . . . . <1.0 d
prepared *(Hunt's Manwich)*, prepared,
   1 sandwich . . . . 2.0 d
Sloppy Joe, dry *(Lawry's* Seasoning Blends),
   1 package . . . . .8 c
Sandwich spread:
meatless, with pickle, 2 tbsp. . . . . .1 d
meatless *(Blue Plate)*, 1 tbsp. 0
meat *(Oscar Mayer)*, 2 oz. 0
Sapodilla:
untrimmed, 1 lb. . . . . 19.2 d
1 medium, 3″ diameter, approximately 7.5 oz.
   untrimmed . . . . 9.0 d
peeled and seeded, ½ cup . . . . 6.4 d
Sapote:
untrimmed, 1 lb. . . . . 8.4 d
1 medium, approximately 11.2 oz. untrimmed . . . 5.9 d
peeled and seeded, 1 oz. . . . . .7 d

Sardines, canned:

in oil, all varieties 0

in tomato sauce, Pacific, drained, 2 oz. . . . . .3 d

in tomato sauce, Pacific, 4 medium, 4¾" long,

    approximately 5.4 oz. . . . . .9 d

Sauce, see specific listings

Sauerkraut, canned:

with liquid, 4 oz. . . . . 2.9 d

with liquid, ½ cup . . . . 3.0 d

(Claussen), 3 oz. . . . . 3.0 d

Sausage:

meat or with cheese, all varieties, 4 oz. 0

"Sausage," imitation:

.9-oz. link . . . . .7 d

1.3-oz. patty . . . . 1.1 d

Sausage seasoning, pork:

(Tone's), 1 tsp. . . . . .7 d

Sausage sticks:

all varieties, 4 oz. 0

Savory, ground:

1 tsp. . . . . .2 c

summer *(Tone's),* 1 tsp. . . . . .2 c

Scallions, see "Onion, spring or green"

Scallops* 0

"Scallop," imitation:

made from surimi 0

Scallop squash:

raw, untrimmed, 1 lb. 8.5 d

raw, trimmed, sliced, ½ cup . . . . 1.2 d

boiled, drained, sliced, ½ cup . . . . 1.1 d

boiled, drained, mashed, ½ cup . . . . 1.4 d

Scotch whiskey:

all varieties 0

Scrod* 0

Scup* 0

Sea bass* 0

Sea trout* 0
Seafood* 0
Seafood seasoning mix:
(Tone's), 1 tsp. . . . . .3 d
Seaweed:
agar, raw, 1 oz. . . . . .1 d
agar, dried, 1 oz. . . . . 2.2 d
Irish moss, raw, 1 oz. .4 d
kelp, raw, 1 oz. . . . . .4 d
laver, raw, 1 oz. . . . . .1 d
spirulina, raw, 1 oz. . . . . .1 c
spirulina, dried, 1 oz. . . . . 1.0 d
wakame, raw, 1 oz. . . . . .1 d
Seltzer:
plain or flavored 0
Semolina:
2 oz. . . . . 2.2 d
½ cup . . . . 3.3 d
Sesame butter, see "Sesame paste" and
  "Tahini"
Sesame flour:
high fat, 1 oz. . . . . 1.8 c
partially defatted, 1 oz. . . . . 1.7 c
low fat, 1 oz. . . . . 1.4 c
Sesame meal:
partially defatted, 1 oz. . . . . 1.1 c
Sesame oil:
all varieties 0
Sesame paste (see also "Tahini"), from whole
  seeds:
1 oz. . . . . 1.6 d
1 tbsp. . . . . .9 d
(Arrowhead Mills), 2 oz. . . . . 3.7 d
Sesame seeds, whole:
dried:
  1 oz. . . . . 3.3 d

Sesame seeds, dried *(cont.)*
½ cup . . . . 8.5 d
1 tbsp. . . . . .1 d
(Arrowhead Mills), 1 oz. . . . . 3.1 d
kernels, toasted, 1 oz. . . . . 4.8 d
roasted and toasted, 1 oz. . . . . 4.0 d
Sesame seeds, dried, decorticated:
1 oz. . . . . .9 d
1 tsp. . . . . .1 d
(Spice Islands), 1 tsp. . . . . .7 c
Sesbania flower:
raw, untrimmed, 1 lb. . . . . 5.8 c
raw, trimmed, 1 cup . . . . .3 c
steamed, ½ cup . . . . .8 c
Shad* 0
Shad roe* 0
Shallots, fresh or stored:
untrimmed, 4 oz. 5.4 c
peeled, 1 oz. . . . . .2 c
chopped, 1 tbsp. .1 c
Shallots, freeze-dried:
1 tbsp. . . . . <.1 c
Shark* 0
Sheepshead* 0
Shellie beans, canned:
with liquid, 4 oz. 3.9 d
with liquid, ½ cup . . . . 4.1 d
Shells, pasta, stuffed, frozen:
(Celentano), 6.25 oz. . . . . 7.0 d
(Celentano Great Choice), 10 oz. . . . . 5.0 d
broccoli *(Celentano* Great Choice), 10 oz. . . . . . 4.0 d
Shells, pasta, mix:
and curry *(Tofu Classics),* prepared, ½ cup . . . . . 3.0 d
Sherbet:
orange, ½ cup . . . . .3 c
bar, orange, 2.75-fl.-oz. bar . . . . .2 c

Shoney's:

soups, 6 oz.:

bean	1.4 d
beef cabbage	2.3 d
broccoli, cream of	.4 d
broccoli-cauliflower	.5 d
cheese Florentine ham	.6 d
chicken, cream of	.3 d
chicken rice	.5 d
onion	.1 d
potato	1.6 d
tomato Florentine	0
tomato vegetable	.4 d
vegetable beef	.3 d

entrees[1], 1 serving:

beef patty, light	0
chicken tenders	0
fish, baked	0
fish, fried, light	.1 d
Fish N'chips, with fries	2.9 d
Fish N'shrimp	.3 d
Italian feast	1.1 d
lasagna	2.8 d
Liver N' Onions	.8 d
seafood platter	.3 d
shrimp, bite-size, boiled, or charbroiled	0
shrimp sampler	.1 d
Shrimper's Feast	.3 d
Shrimper's Feast, large	.4 d
spaghetti	2.2 d
steak, country fried	.9 d
steak, rib eye or sirloin	0
Steak N'shrimp, fried shrimp	.1 d
Steak N'shrimp, charbroiled shrimp	0

---

[1] Does not include potato, bread, or salad bar.

Shoney's (cont.)

burgers, 1 serving:
All-American or bacon . . . . .5 d
mushroom-Swiss . . . . .7 d
Old-Fashioned . . . . .6 d
Shoney . . . . .2 d

sandwiches, 1 serving:
bacon & cheese, grilled . . . . 1.3 d
cheese, grilled . . . . 1.4 d
chicken, fillet or charbroiled . . . . .5 d
country fried . . . . 1.4 d
fish . . . . .4 d
ham, baked . . . . 1.8 d
ham club, whole wheat . . . . 10.2 d
Patty Melt . . . . 6.7 d
Philly steak . . . . .1 d
Reuben . . . . 6.3 d
Slim Jim . . . . .5 d
turkey club, whole wheat . . . . 10.2 d

side dishes, 1 serving:
mushrooms, sauteed . . . . 1.3 d
onions, sautéed . . . . .5 d
onion rings, 1 piece . . . . .4 d
potato, baked, 10 oz. . . . . 6.8 d
french fries, 3 oz. . . . . 2.7 d
french fries, 4 oz. . . . . 3.6 d
rice . . . . .1 d

salads, prepared, ¼ cup:
ambrosia . . . . .8 d
apple-grape surprise . . . . .1 d
beet onion . . . . .8 d
broccoli/cauliflower . . . . .9 d
broccoli/cauliflower/carrot or ranch . . . . .9 d
carrot apple or coleslaw . . . . .9 d
cucumber lite . . . . .2 d
fruit, glaced . . . . .5 d

fruit, mixed	.2 d
fruit delight	.7 d
kidney bean	1.9 d
macaroni	.2 d
Oriental	.5 d
pasta, Don's, rotelli, or spaghetti	.2 d
pea	2.4 d
Seigan	1.2 d
snow	.1 d
spring	.7 d
squash, mixed	.3 d
summer	.9 d
three bean	1.3 d
vegetable, Italian	.7 d
Waldorf	.8 d
dressings, all varieties, 2 tbsp.	0
sauce, BBQ, cocktail, sweet 'n sour, or tartar, 1 soufflé cup	0

desserts, 1 serving:

hot fudge sundae	0
strawberry pie	2.3 d
strawberry sundae	.3 d

Short ribs* 0

Shortening:

all varieties and blends 0

Shoyu, see "Soy sauce"

Shrimp* 0

"Shrimp," imitation:

made from surimi 0

Shrimp chow mein, canned:

(La Choy), 3/4 cup	2.0 d
(La Choy) Bi-Pack), 3/4 cup	1.0 d

Shrimp cocktail:

(Sau-Sea), 4-oz. jar	3.0 d
(Sau-Sea), 6-oz. jar	4.0 d

Shrimp Creole mix, dry:
(Luzianne), 1/5 package . . . . <1.0 d
Shrimp and okra gumbo, frozen:
(Bodin's), 4 oz. . . . . 1.0 d
Shrimp spice:
(Tone's Craboil), 1 tsp. . . . . .3 d
Skipjack* 0
Skunk cabbage, see "Swamp cabbage"
Sloppy Joe sauce, see "Sandwich sauce"
Sloppy Joe seasoning, see "Sandwich
  seasoning mix"
Smelt* 0
Snack bars (see also "Granola and cereal
  bars"):
all varieties *(Health Valley Fat Free Bakes),*
  1 bar . . . . 2.5 d
all varieties *(Health Valley Fat Free Fruit Bars),*
  1 bar . . . . 3.7 d
Snack mix, 1 oz.:
(Flavor House Party Mix), 1 oz. . . . . 2.0 d
(Pepperidge Farm Classic/Goldfish Party Mix),
  1 oz. . . . . 1.0 d
lightly smoked, zesty herb, or spicy
  (Pepperidge Farm), 1 oz. . . . . 1.0 d
nutty *(Pepperidge Farm),* 1 oz. . . . . 2.0 d
Snails* 0
Snap beans, see "Green beans"
Snapper* 0
Snow peas, see "Peas, edible-podded"
Snow pea mix, Oriental:
with rice *(Fantastic),* prepared, 10 oz. . . . . 3.0 d
Soft drinks, carbonated:
all varieties 0
Sole* 0
Sorghum:
whole grain, 1 cup . . . . 4.6 c

Sorghum syrup:

1 fl. oz. 0

Sorrel, see "Dock"

Soup, canned, ready-to-serve:

bean *(Grandma Brown's),* 1 cup . . . . 9.8 d

bean, black:

   (Hain 99% Fat Free), 9.5 oz. . . . . 10.5 d

   (Progresso Hearty), 9.5 oz. . . . . 11.0 d

   and carrots *(Health Valley* Fat Free), 7.5 oz. . . . 17.0 d

bean, with ham, 1 cup . . . . 11.2 d

beef, chunky, 1 cup . . . . 1.4 d

beef barley *(Progresso),* 9.5 oz. . . . . 4.0 d

beef bouillon, broth, or consommé, 1 cup 0

chicken:

   chunky, 1 cup . . . . 1.5 d

   barley *(Progresso),* 9.25 oz. . . . . 4.0 d

   broth or consommé, 1 cup 0

   noodle, chunky, 1 cup . . . . 3.8 d

   rice, chunky, 1 cup . . . . 1.0 d

clam chowder, Manhattan, 1 cup . . . . 2.9 d

corn and vegetable, country *(Health Valley* Fat

   Free), 7.5 oz. . . . . 3.0 d

crab, 1 cup . . . . .7 d

gazpacho, 1 cup . . . . 3.7 d

ham and bean *(Progresso),* 9.5 oz. . . . . 10.0 d

lentil:

   (Progresso), 9.5 oz. . . . . 7.0 d

   and carrots *(Health Valley* Fat Free), 7.5 oz. . . . 15.0 d

   with sausage *(Progresso),* 9.5 oz. . . . . 5.0 d

   vegetarian *(Hain* 99% Fat Free), 9.5 oz. . . . . . . 5.5 d

macaroni and bean *(Progresso),* 9.5 oz. . . . . 6.5 d

minestrone:

   (Health Valley), 7.5 oz. . . . . 5.8 d

   (Progresso), 9.5 oz. . . . . 7.0 d

   hearty or zesty *(Progresso),* 9.25 oz. . . . . 4.0 d

   real Italian *(Health Valley* Fat Free), 7.5 oz. . . . . 4.0 d

Soup, canned, ready-to-serve *(cont.)*
pea, split:

   (Grandma Brown's), 1 cup . . . .   5.8 d

   and carrots *(Health Valley* Fat Free), 7.5 oz. . . .   12.5 d

   green *(Progresso),* 9.5 oz. . . . .   5.0 d

   with ham *(Progresso),* 9.5 oz. . . . .   6.0 d

   vegetarian *(Hain* 99% Fat Free), 9.5 oz. . . . . . .   4.0 d

tomato *(Progresso),* 9.5 oz. . . . .   4.0 d

tomato vegetable *(Health Valley* Fat Free),

   7.5 oz. . . . .   3.0 d

tortellini *(Progresso),* 9.5 oz. . . . .   2.0 d

vegetable:

   (Progresso), 9.5 oz.   3.0 d

   14 garden or 5 bean *(Health Valley* Fat Free),

      7.5 oz. . . . .   3.0 d

   barley *(Health Valley* Fat Free), 7.5 oz. . . . .   4.0 d

   with pasta *(Progresso* Hearty), 9.5 oz. . . . .   4.0 d

wild rice *(Hain* 99% Fat Free), 9.5 oz. . . . .   3.0 d

Soup, canned, condensed[1]:

asparagus, cream of, 1 cup . . . .   .5 d

barley and bean *(Rokeach),* 1 cup . . . .   5.0 d

bean:

   (Campbell's Homestyle), 8 oz. . . . .   6.0 d

   black, 1 cup . . . .   8.4 d

   with bacon *(Campbell's/Campbell's* Healthy

      Request), 8 oz. . . . .   6.0 d

   with frankfurters, 1 cup . . . .   5.8 d

   with pork, 1 cup . . . .   7.5 d

beef bouillon, broth, or consommé, 1 cup   0

beef noodle, 1 cup . . . .   1.5 d

celery, cream of, 1 cup . . . .   .7 d

cheese, 1 cup . . . .   1.0 d

chicken:

   broth, bouillon, or consommé, 1 cup   0

---

[1] Diluted according to label directions, with equal amounts of water and/or milk.

cream of, 1 cup .... .2 d
with dumplings, 1 cup .... .7 d
gumbo, 1 cup .... 2.0 d
mushroom, 1 cup .... .3 d
noodle, 1 cup .... .7 d
with rice, 1 cup .... .6 d
vegetable, 1 cup .... 1.0 d
chili beef, 1 cup .... 9.0 d
clam chowder, Manhattan, 1 cup .... 1.5 d
clam chowder, New England, 1 cup .... .7 d
minestrone, 1 cup .... 1.0 d
mushroom:
  barley, 1 cup............................ .7 d
  with beef stock, 1 cup.................. .1 d
  cream of, 1 cup .... .4 d
onion, 1 cup .... .8 d
onion, cream of, 1 cup .... .5 d
oyster stew, 1 cup 0
pea:
  green *(Campbell's),* 8 oz. .... 4.0 d
  split *(Rokeach),* 1 cup .... 4.0 d
  split, with ham and bacon *(Campbell's),* 8 oz. . 4.0 d
potato, cream of, 1 cup .... .5 d
shrimp, cream of, 1 cup .... .2 d
tomato:
  1 cup .... .5 d
  beef, with noodle, 1 cup .... 1.5 d
  with rice, 1 cup .... 1.5 d
  with rice *(Rokeach),* 1 cup .... 2.0 d
turkey noodle, 1 cup .... .7 d
turkey vegetable, 1 cup .... .5 d
vegetable *(Rokeach),* 1 cup .... 3.0 d
vegetable beef, 1 cup .... 1.9 d

Soup mix, prepared, except as noted:

barley, better *(Aunt Patsy's* Pantry), 8 oz. . . . . . . 5.0 d

barley vegetable *(Fantastic Bouncin' Barley*
  Vegetable), 10 oz. . . . . 8.0 d

bean:

  black *(Fantastic Jumpin' Black Beans),* 10 oz. . 13.0 d

  many *(Aunt Patsy's* Pantry), 8 oz. . . . . 4.0 d

  navy *(Aunt Patsy's* Pantry), 8 oz. . . . . 3.0 d

  7, and barley *(Arrowhead Mills),* 1 oz. dry . . . . 12.5 d

beef bouillon, broth or consommé, 1 cup 0

beef noodle, 1 cup . . . . .8 d

broccoli, in cheddar *(Fantastic Dancin'*
  Broccoli), 10 oz. . . . . 2.0 d

broccoli and cheese *(Lipton Cup-a-Soup),*
  6 fl. oz. . . . . 1.0 d

chicken:

  bouillon, broth, or consommé, 1 cup 0

  cream of, 1 cup . . . . .3 d

  flavor, thyme *(Aunt Patsy's* Pantry), 8 oz. . . . . . 2.0 d

  rice, 1 cup . . . . .8 d

  vegetable, creamy *(Lipton Cup-a-Soup),*
    1 pouch . . . . 1.0 d

corn and potato chowder *(Fantastic Jammin'),*
  10 oz. . . . . 2.0 d

leek, 1 cup . . . . 3.0 d

lentil *(Fantastic Laughin' Lentils),* 10 oz. . . . . 12.0 d

lentil, red *(Aunt Patsy's* Pantry), 8 oz. . . . . 3.0 d

minestrone, with pasta *(Fantastic Serandin'*
  Minestrone), 10 oz. 5.0 d

mushroom, cream of *(Fantastic Marchin' Cream*
  of Mushroom), 10 oz. . . . . 2.0 d

mushroom, creamy *(Lipton Cup-a-Soup),*
  6 fl. oz. . . . . <1.0 d

noodle:

  beef or chicken *(La Choy),* 1 cup . . . . 4.0 d

beef or chicken *(Maruchan* Instant Picante),
   2.25 oz. dry . . . . 3.0 d
cheddar, creamy *(Fantastic Noodles),* 7 oz. . . . 2.5 d
curry vegetable *(Fantastic Noodles),* 7 oz. . . . . 3.2 d
miso vegetable *(Fantastic Noodles),* 7 oz. . . . . 3.0 d
shrimp *(Maruchan* Instant Picante), 2.25 oz.
   dry . . . . 4.0 d
tomato vegetable *(Fantastic Noodles),* 7 oz. . . . 3.2 d
vegetable, California *(Maruchan* Instant
   Picante), 2.25 oz. dry . . . . 4.0 d
whole wheat *(Fantastic Rockin' ABC's),*
   10 oz. . . . . 4.0 d
oxtail, 1 cup . . . . .5 d
pea:
   green *(Lipton Cup-a-Soup),* 6 fl. oz. . . . . 2.0 d
   plentiful *(Aunt Patsy's* Pantry), 8 oz. . . . . 6.0 d
   split *(Fantastic Splittin' Peas),* 10 oz. . . . . 10.0 d
   Virginia *(Lipton Cup-a-Soup),* 6 fl. oz. . . . . 3.0 d
tomato or tomato vegetable, 1 cup . . . . .5 d
tomato *(Lipton Cup-a-Soup),* 6 fl. oz. . . . . 1.0 d
vegetable:
   country *(Lipton* Cook Up), 1 cup . . . . 2.0 d
   harvest *(Lipton Cup-a-Soup* Hearty), 6 fl. oz. . 2.0 d
   spring *(Lipton Cup-a-Soup),* 6 fl. oz. . . . . <1.0 d
Sour cream:
dairy or nondairy 0
Soursop:
untrimmed, 1 lb. . . . . 10.0 d
1 medium, approximately 2 lbs. untrimmed . . . . . 20.6 d
peeled and seeded, ½ cup . . . . 3.7 d
Souse loaf:
all varieties, 4 oz. 0
Soy beans, see "Soybeans"
Soy beverage:
(Soy Moo Fat Free), 8 fl. oz. 0

Soy flour:
(Arrowhead Mills), 2 oz. . . . .   8.1 d
full fat, raw, 2 oz. . . . .   5.5 d
full fat, raw, ½ cup stirred . . . .   4.0 d
defatted, 2 oz. . . . .   10.0 d
defatted, ½ cup stirred . . . .   8.8 d
low fat, 2 oz. . . . .   5.8 d
low fat, ½ cup stirred . . . .   4.5 d
Soy meal:
defatted, raw, ½ cup . . . .   7.0 d
Soy milk, fluid:
8 fl. oz. . . . .   3.1 d
Soy protein:
concentrate, 1 oz.   1.1 c
Soy sauce:
(La Choy/La Choy Lite), ½ tsp. . . . .   <1.0 d
tamari or shoyu, 1 tbsp. . . . .   .1 d
tamari or shoyu *(Eden/Eden Naturally Brewed)*,
  ½ tsp.   0
Soybean cake or curd, see "Tofu"
Soybean flakes:
(Arrowhead Mills), 2 oz. . . . .   8.1 d
Soybean kernels, raw and toasted:
1 oz., approximately 95 kernels . . . .   1.0 d
whole, ½ cup . . . .   1.9 d
Soybean (soya) oil:
all varieties   0
Soybeans, fermented, see "Miso" and
  "Natto"
Soybeans, green:
raw, in pods, 1 lb.   10.1 d
raw, shelled, ½ cup . . . .   5.4 d
boiled, drained, ½ cup . . . .   3.8 d
Soybeans, mature, dry:
raw:
  1 oz. . . . .   2.6 d

½ cup . . . . 8.6 d
(Arrowhead Mills), 2 oz. . . . . 13.2 d
boiled, ½ cup . . . . 5.2 d
dry-roasted, 1 oz. 2.3 d
dry-roasted, ½ cup . . . . 7.0 d
Soybeans, sprouted, mature seeds:
raw, 4 oz. . . . . 2.6 c
raw, ½ cup . . . . .8 c
steamed, ½ cup . . . . .4 d
stir-fried, 4 oz. . . . . 2.9 c
Spaghetti, see "Pasta"
Spaghetti dishes, mix:
whole wheat *(Fantastic All-O-Round)*, prepared,
  10 oz. . . . . 5.0 d
Spaghetti sauce, see "Pasta sauce" and
  specific listings
Spaghetti squash:
raw, untrimmed, 1 lb. . . . . 4.8 d
raw, cubed, ½ cup .8 d
baked or boiled and drained, ½ cup . . . . 1.1 d
Spareribs* 0
Spelt flakes:
(Arrowhead Mills), 1 oz. . . . . 3.0 d
Spelt flour:
(Arrowhead Mills), 2 oz. . . . . 8.0 d
Spice loaf:
(Kahn's), 2 oz. 0
Spinach, fresh:
raw:
  untrimmed, 1 lb. 8.8 d
  trimmed, 10-oz. package . . . . 7.7 d
  trimmed, chopped, ½ cup . . . . .8 d
boiled, drained, ½ cup . . . . 2.2 d
Spinach, canned:
with liquid, 4 oz. . . . . 2.5 d
with liquid, ½ cup . . . . 2.6 d

Spinach, canned *(cont.)*
drained, 4 oz. . . . . 2.7 d
drained, ½ cup . . . . 2.6 d
Spinach, frozen:
chopped or leaf:
   unheated, 3.3 oz. 2.8 d
   unheated, ½ cup . . . . 2.3 d
   boiled, drained, ½ cup . . . . 2.6 d
(Green Giant), ½ cup . . . . 5.0 d
(Green Giant Harvest Fresh), ½ cup . . . . 3.0 d
creamed *(Birds Eye),* 3 oz. . . . . 1.0 d
creamed *(Green Giant),* ½ cup . . . . 2.0 d
in butter sauce, cut *(Green Giant),* ½ cup . . . . . 3.5 d
Spinach, New Zealand, see "New Zealand
  spinach"
Spiny lobster* 0
Spirulina, see "Seaweed"
Split peas, dry:
raw, 1 oz. . . . . 7.2 d
raw, ½ cup . . . . 25.1 d
boiled, ½ cup . . . . 8.1 d
green *(Arrowhead Mills),* 2 oz. . . . . 7.5 d
Spot:
all varieties* 0
Spring onion, see "Onion, spring or green"
Sprouts (see also specific listings):
bean, canned *(La Choy),* ⅔ cup . . . . <1.0 d
mixed *(Shaw's Premium),* 2 oz. . . . . 2.0 d
Squab* 0
Squash, see specific listings
Squash seeds, see "Pumpkin seed kernels"
Squid* 0
Star fruit, see "Carambola"
Steak:
meat, poultry, or fish* 0

Steak, pepper, entree:

canned *(La Choy* Bi-Pack), ¾ cup . . . .   2.0 d

canned, Oriental *(La Choy),* ¾ cup . . . .   2.0 d

mi *(La Choy* Dinner Classics), prepared, ¾ cup . . .   1.0 d

Steak sauce:

(Lea & Perrins), 1 tbsp.   0

(Maull's), 1 tbsp.   0

regular or hickory smoke *(Heinz 57),* 1 tbsp.   0

Straightneck squash, fresh:

raw, untrimmed, 1 lb. . . . .   8.2 d

raw, trimmed, sliced, ½ cup . . . .   1.2 d

boiled, drained, ½ cup . . . .   1.3 d

Straightneck squash, canned:

with liquid, 4 oz. or ½ cup . . . .   1.1 d

Straightneck squash, frozen:

unheated, 3.3 oz. . . . .   1.1 d

unheated, ½ cup . . . .   .8 d

boiled, sliced, ½ cup . . . .   1.2 d

Stomach, pork*   0

Strawberries, fresh:

1 pint . . . .   7.4 d

4 oz. . . . .   2.6 d

½ cup . . . .   1.7 d

Strawberries, canned, in syrup:

4 oz. . . . .   1.9 d

½ cup . . . .   2.2 d

Strawberries, frozen:

unsweetened, 5 oz. . . . .   3.0 d

unsweetened, ½ cup . . . .   1.6 d

sweetened, 5 oz. . . . .   2.2 d

sweetened, whole, ½ cup . . . .   2.4 d

frozen in syrup *(Birds Eye* Lite), 5 oz. . . . .   2.0 d

Strawberry cobbler, see "Cobbler, frozen"

Strawberry flavor drink mix:

2–3 heaping tsp., approximately ¾ oz. . . . .   <.1 d

(Kool-Aid), 8 fl. oz.   0

Strawberry milk drink:

chilled *(Nestlé Quik)*, 1 cup . . . .   (0)

mix, powder, 1 oz. dry . . . .   <.1 c

Strawberry pie, see "Pie"

Strawberry supreme torte, see "Cake"

String beans, see "Green beans"

Stroganoff, vegetarian, see "Vegetable

 Stroganoff mix"

Stroganoff sauce mix:

(Lawry's), 1 package . . . .   .8 c

Stuffing:

bread, mix, ½ cup prepared . . . .   1.5 d

corn *(Arnold)*, 1 oz. . . . .   2.0 d

cornbread *(Brownberry)*, 1 oz. . . . .   2.0 d

cube, unspiced *(Arnold)*, ½ oz. . . . .   1.0 d

herb seasoned or sage and onion

 (Arnold/Brownberry), ½ oz. . . . .   1.0 d

sage and onion *(Pepperidge Farm* Distinctive),

 1 oz. . . . .   2.0 d

seasoned *(Arnold)*, ½ oz. . . . .   1.0 d

Sturgeon*   0

Succotash, fresh:

boiled, drained, ½ cup . . . .   1.3 c

Succotash, canned:

with whole kernel corn, 4 oz. . . . .   6.2 d

with whole kernel corn, ½ cup . . . .   6.9 d

with cream-style corn, ½ cup . . . .   1.7 c

Succotash, frozen:

boiled, drained, 4 oz. . . . .   6.2 d

boiled, drained, ½ cup . . . .   4.6 d

Sucker*   0

Sugar, beet or cane:

all varieties   0

Sugar, maple:

1 oz. 0

Sugar, substitute:

(Equal), 1 packet 0

(NutraSweet), 1 tsp. 0

Sugar apple:

untrimmed, 1 lb. . . . . 11.0 d

1 medium, 2⅞" diameter, approximately 9.9 oz.
  untrimmed . . . . 6.8 d

peeled and seeded, ½ cup . . . . 5.5 d

Sugar snap peas, see "Peas, edible-podded"

Summer sausage:

all varieties, 4 oz. 0

Summer squash (see also specific squash
  listings), fresh:

untrimmed, 1 lb. . . . . 8.2 d

trimmed, sliced, ½ cup . . . . 1.2 d

boiled, drained, sliced, ½ cup . . . . 1.3 d

Sunfish* 0

Sunflower seed butter:

1 oz. . . . . 1.4 d

1 tbsp. . . . . .8 d

Sunflower seed flour, partially defatted:

4 oz. . . . . 5.9 d

1 cup . . . . 4.2 d

1 tbsp. . . . . .3 d

Sunflower seed oil:

all varieties 0

Sunflower seeds, kernels:

(Arrowhead Mills), 1 oz. . . . . 4.4 d

dried, 1 oz. . . . . 3.0 d

dried, ½ cup . . . . 7.6 d

dry-roasted:

  1 oz. . . . . 2.6 d

  ½ cup . . . . 5.8 d

Sunflower seeds, dry-roasted *(cont.)*
  (Fisher), 1 oz. . . . . 5.0 d
  (Flavor House), 1 oz. . . . . 3.0 d
oil-roasted, 1 oz. . . . . 1.9 d
oil-roasted, 1/2 cup . . . . 4.6 d
Surimi:
made from walleye pollack 0
Swamp cabbage:
raw, untrimmed, 1 lb. 7.3 d
raw, 1 shoot, approximately .6 oz. untrimmed . . . . .3 d
boiled, drained, chopped, 1/2 cup . . . . .9 d
Sweet peas, see "Green peas"
Sweet potato, fresh:
raw, untrimmed, 1 lb. 9.8 d
raw, 1 medium, 5″ × 2″ diameter, approximately
  6.3 oz. untrimmed . . . . 3.9 d
baked in skin, 1 medium, 5″ × 2″ . . . . 3.4 d
baked in skin, mashed, 1/2 cup . . . . 3.0 d
boiled without skin, 4 oz. . . . . 2.8 d
boiled, without skin, mashed, 1/2 cup . . . . 4.1 d
Sweet potato, canned:
in syrup:
  with liquid, 4 oz. . . . . 2.1 d
  with liquid, 1/2 cup . . . . 2.1 d
  drained, 1/2 cup . . . . 1.8 d
vacuum pack:
  4 oz. . . . . 3.4 d
  pieces, 1/2 cup . . . . 3.0 d
  mashed, 1/2 cup . . . . 3.8 d
Sweet potato, frozen:
baked, 4 oz. . . . . 3.4 d
baked, cubed, 1/2 cup . . . . 2.6 d
patty *(Stilwell* Yam Patties), 2 pieces . . . . 3.0 d
Sweet potato leaf:
raw, chopped, 1/2 cup . . . . .2 c
steamed, 1/2 cup . . . . .6 d

Sweet and sour cocktail mixer:
bottled, 3 fl. oz. . . . . (0)
Sweet and sour sauce:
(La Choy/La Choy Duck Sauce), 1 tbsp. . . . . <1.0 d
(Woody's), 2 tbsp. . . . . <1.0 d
Sweetbreads* 0
Sweetsop, see "Sugar apple"
Swiss chard:
raw:
  untrimmed, 1 lb. . . . . 6.7 d
  1 leaf, approximately 1.7 oz. . . . . .8 d
  chopped, ½ cup . . . . .3 d
boiled, drained, chopped, ½ cup . . . . 1.8 d
Swordfish* 0
Syrup, see specific listings
Szechwan sauce:
(La Choy), 1 oz. 0

T

Food and Measure

Fiber Grams

Tabbouleh mix, prepared *(Fantastic)*, ½ cup . . . .   5.0 d
Taco mix:
(Tio Sancho Dinner Kit):
    sauce, 2 oz. . . . .   .5 c
    seasoning, 1.25 oz. . . . .   1.7 c
    shell . . . .   .5 c
Taco sauce:
(Lawry's Sauce'n Seasoner), ¼ cup   0
(Old El Paso), 2 tbsp. . . . .   1.0 d
chunky *(Lawry's)*, ¼ cup . . . .   .4 c
Taco seasoning mix, dry:
(Lawry's Seasoning Blends), 1.25 oz. . . . .   1.0 c
(Tio Sancho), 1.51 oz. . . . .   2.0 c
salad *(Lawry's* Seasoning Blends), 1 package . . .   1.6 c
Taco shell:
(Gebhardt), 1 piece . . . .   <1.0 d
(Lawry's), 1 piece . . . .   .2 c
(Lawry's Super), 1 piece . . . .   .4 c
(Old El Paso), 1 piece . . . .   .5 d
(Old El Paso Super), 1 piece . . . .   1.5 d
(Rosarita), 1 piece . . . .   <1.0 d
(Tio Sancho), 1 piece . . . .   .5 c
(Tio Sancho Super), 1 piece . . . .   .7 c
mini *(Old El Paso)*, 3 pieces . . . .   .5 d

Tahini:

all varieties, 1 oz.	2.6 d
from unroasted kernels, 1 tbsp.	1.3 d
from roasted and toasted kernels, 1 tbsp.	1.4 d
(Arrowhead Mills), 1 oz.	2.6 d
imported (Krinos), 1 oz.	2.0 d

Tallow:

all varieties	0

Tamale, canned:

(Derby), 2 pieces	1.0 d
(Gebhardt), 2 pieces	2.0 d
(Gebhardt Jumbo), 2 pieces	3.0 d

Tamari, see "Soy sauce"

Tamarind:

untrimmed, 1 lb.	7.9 d
10 medium, 3″ long, approximately 2.1 oz. untrimmed	1.0 d
trimmed, ½ cup	3.1 d

Tangerine, fresh:

untrimmed, 1 lb.	7.5 d
1 medium, 2⅜″ diameter, approximately 4.2 oz. untrimmed	1.9 d
sections without membrane, ½ cup	2.2 d

Tangerine, canned (Mandarin orange):

in juice or syrup, 4 oz.	.8 d
in juice or syrup, ½ cup	.9 d

Tangerine juice:

fresh, canned, or frozen and diluted, 6 fl. oz.	.4 d
frozen concentrate, undiluted, 6 fl. oz.	1.3 d

Tapioca, pearl, dry:

2 oz.	.5 d
½ cup	1.4 d
1 tbsp.	.2 d

Taramasalata (Krinos) | 0

Taro:
raw, untrimmed, 1 lb. . . . . 16.0 d
raw, sliced, ½ cup . . . . 2.1 d
cooked, 4 oz. . . . . 5.8 d
cooked, sliced, ½ cup . . . . 3.4 d
Taro chips:
1 oz. . . . . .3 c
½ cup . . . . .1 c
Taro leaf:
raw:
  untrimmed, 1 lb. 10.1 d
  1 leaf, approximately .3 oz. untrimmed . . . . . . .4 d
  trimmed, ½ cup . . . . .5 d
steamed, ½ cup . . . . .4 c
Taro shoots:
raw, sliced, ½ cup .3 c
cooked, sliced, ½ cup . . . . .4 c
Taro, Tahitian:
raw, sliced, ½ cup . . . . 1.1 c
cooked, sliced, ½ cup . . . . 1.6 c
Tarragon, ground:
1 oz. . . . . 2.1 d
1 tsp. . . . . .1 d
Tart shell, see "Pastry dough"
Tartar sauce:
(Lyon/Lyon Lite), 1 tbsp. 0
Tautog* 0
Tea:
regular, instant, or herbal, 8 fl. oz. 0
Tea, iced:
canned, instant, or mix, plain or flavored,
  8 fl. oz. 0
Teff seed:
(Arrowhead Mills), 2 oz. . . . . 7.7 d
Teff flour:
(Arrowhead Mills), 2 oz. . . . . 7.7 d

Tempeh:
1 oz. . . . . .8 c
½ cup . . . . 2.5 c
Tendergreens, see "Mustard spinach"
Tequila:
all varieties 0
Teriyaki marinade:
(Lawry's), 2 tbsp. .2 c
barbecue *(Lawry's),* ¼ cup . . . . .2 c
Teriyaki sauce:
all varieties *(La Choy),* ½ tsp. . . . . <1.0 d
Thuringer cervelat:
all varieties, 4 oz. 0
Thyme, ground:
1 oz. . . . . 5.3 d
1 tsp. . . . . .3 d
Thymus* 0
Tilefish* 0
Toaster muffins and pastries:
apple cinnamon *(Kellogg's Pop-Tarts),* 1 piece . . .   1.0 d
banana nut *(Thomas' Toast-r-Cakes),* 1 piece . . .   1.0 d
blueberry *(Thomas' Toast-r-Cakes),* 1 piece . . . . . <1.0 d
blueberry, plain or frosted *(Kellogg's Pop-Tarts),*
    1 piece 0
brown sugar–cinnamon, plain or frosted
    (Kellogg's Pop-Tarts), 1 piece 0
cherry, plain or frosted *(Kellogg's Pop-Tarts),*
    1 piece 0
chocolate chip *(Thomas' Toast-r-Cakes),*
    1 piece . . . . 2.0 d
chocolate fudge or chocolate-vanilla creme,
    frosted *(Kellogg's Pop-Tarts),* 1 piece 0
chocolate graham *(Kellogg's Pop-Tarts),* 1 piece   0
corn *(Thomas' Toast-r-Cakes),* 1 piece . . . . <1.0 d
grape or raspberry, frosted *(Kellogg's Pop-
    Tarts),* 1 piece 0

Toaster muffins and pastries *(cont.)*

oat bran with raisins *(Awrey's Toastums)*,
1 piece . . . .   1.0 d

oat bran with raisins *(Thomas' Toast-r-Cakes)*,
1 piece . . . .   1.0 d

strawberry *(Kellogg's Pop-Tarts)*, 1 piece   0

strawberry, frosted *(Kellogg's Pop-Tarts)*,
1 piece . . . .   1.0 d

Tofu:

raw, regular:

   1 oz. . . . .   .3 d

   ¼ block, approximately 4.1 oz. . . . .   1.4 d

   ½ cup . . . .   1.5 d

raw, firm:

   1 oz. . . . .   .7 d

   ¼ block, approximately 2.9 oz. . . . .   1.9 d

   ½ cup . . . .   2.9 d

dried-frozen (koyadofu), 1 oz. . . . .   <.1 c

fried, 1 oz. . . . .   1.1 d

okara, 1 oz. . . . .   1.2 c

okara, ½ cup . . . .   2.5 c

salted and fermented (fuyu), 1 oz. . . . .   .1 c

Tomatillo:

4 oz. . . . .   2.2 d

1 medium, 1⅝″ diameter, approximately 1.2 oz. . . .   .6 d

chopped, ½ cup . . . .   1.3 d

Tomato, fresh, red (see also "Tomato, green"):

raw:

   untrimmed, 1 lb. . . . .   4.5 d

   1 medium, 2⅗″ diameter, approximately
      4.8 oz. untrimmed . . . .   1.4 d

   trimmed, chopped, ½ cup . . . .   1.0 d

boiled, ½ cup . . . .   1.2 d

stewed, seasoned, ½ cup . . . .   .9 d

Tomato, canned (see also "Tomato sauce"):
whole:

4 oz.	1.1 d
½ cup	.6 d
(Del Monte), ½ cup	2.0 d
all varieties *(Hunt's)*, 4 oz.	<1.0 d

cut, peeled *(Hunt's* Choice Cut), 4 oz. . . . . 1.0 d
diced, in tomato juice *(Del Monte)*, ½ cup . . . . . 2.0 d
crushed *(Hunt's* Angela Mia/*Hunt's* Italian
   Flavored), 4 oz. . . . . <1.0 d
with jalapeños *(Old El Paso)*, ¼ cup 0
paste, see "Tomato paste"
puree:

4 oz.	2.6 d
½ cup	2.9 d
(Del Monte), ¼ cup	1.0 d
(Hunt's), 4 oz.	2.0 d

stewed:

½ cup	.9 d
(Del Monte/Del Monte No Salt Added), ½ cup	2.0 d
(Hunt's/Hunt's No Salt Added), 4 oz.	<1.0 d
Italian flavored *(Hunt's)*, 4 oz.	<1.0 d

  Italian, Mexican, or pizza style *(Del Monte)*,
    ½ cup . . . . 2.0 d
wedges *(Del Monte)*, ½ cup . . . . 2.0 d
wedges, in tomato juice, ½ cup . . . . .6 c
Tomato, dried, see "Tomato, sun-dried"
Tomato, green, fresh:
untrimmed, 1 lb. . . . . 6.2 d
1 medium, 2⅗" diameter, approximately 4.8 oz.
  untrimmed . . . . 1.8 d
Tomato, green, pickled:
(Claussen), 3 oz. . . . . 2.0 d

Tomato, sun-dried, dry:

4 oz. . . . . 14.0 d
10 pieces, approximately .7 oz. . . . . 2.5 d
½ cup, approximately 16 pieces . . . . 3.3 d
Tomato juice:
regular, 6 fl. oz. . . . . .7 d
low sodium, 6 fl. oz. 1.5 d
(Campbell's), 6 fl. oz. . . . . 1.0 d
(Hunt's/Hunt's No Salt Added), 6 fl. oz. . . . . 2.0 d
Tomato paste:
6-oz. can . . . . 7.5 d
1 oz. . . . . 1.2 d
¼ cup . . . . 2.9 d
1 tbsp. . . . . .7 d
(Del Monte), 2 tbsp. 2.0 d
(Hunt's/Hunt's No Salt Added), 2 oz. . . . . 2.0 d
Italian or with garlic *(Hunt's),* 2 oz. . . . . 2.0 d
Tomato puree, see "Tomato, canned"
Tomato sauce, canned (see also "Tomato,
    canned"):
4 oz. . . . . 1.6 d
½ cup . . . . 1.7 d
(Del Monte), ¼ cup 0
(Hunt's/Hunt's No Salt/Special), 4 oz. . . . . 2.0 d
Italian style, herb flavored, or with garlic
    (Hunt's), 4 oz. . . . . 2.0 d
marinara, ½ cup . . . . .8 c
for meatloaf *(Hunt's Meatloaf Fixin's),* 2 oz. . . . . . <1.0 d
with mushrooms *(Rokeach),* 1 cup . . . . 6.0 d
with mushrooms, onions, or tomato bits
    (Hunt's), 4 oz. . . . . 2.0 d
with onion, green pepper, and celery, 4 oz. . . . . . 3.9 d
with onion, green pepper, and celery, ½ cup . . . 4.1 d
pasta, see "Pasta sauce"
pizza, see "Pizza sauce"
Tongue* 0

Tortellini Provençale, frozen:
(Green Giant Garden Gourmet Right for Lunch),
  9.5 oz. . . . . 3.0 d
Tortilla chips:
plain, 1 oz. . . . . 1.9 d
(NaChips), 1 oz. . . . . 1.5 d
all varieties *(Doritos)*, 1 oz. . . . . 1.5 d
all varieties *(Tostitos)*, 1 oz. . . . . 1.5 d
blue *(Kettle Tias* Lightly Salted/No Salt), 1 oz. . . . 2.0 d
Tortilla mix:
corn *(Albers Ricamasa)*, ⅓ cup . . . . 5.0 d
Tortilla shell:
corn, 1 medium, 6″ to 7″ diameter,
  approximately .9 oz. . . . . 1.3 d
flour, 1 medium, 7″ to 8″ diameter,
  approximately 1.2 oz. . . . . 1.1 d
Tostaco shell:
(Old El Paso), 1 piece . . . . 1.0 d
Tostada shell:
(Lawry's), 1 piece . . . . .4 d
(Old El Paso), 1 piece . . . . .5 d
(Rosarita), 1 piece . . . . <1.0 d
(Tio Sancho), 1 piece . . . . .5 c
Tree fern, cooked:
4 oz. . . . . 4.2 d
chopped, ½ cup . . . . 2.6 d
Triticale, whole grain:
2 oz. . . . . 10.3 d
½ cup . . . . 17.4 d
Triticale flour, whole grain:
2 oz. . . . . 8.3 d
½ cup . . . . 9.5 d
Trout* 0
Tuna* 0
Tuna, canned in oil 0

Tuna salad spread:
(*Libby's Spreadables*), 1.9 oz. . . . . 1.0 d
Turbot* 0
Turkey* 0
Turkey bacon:
all varieties, 4 oz. 0
Turkey bologna:
all varieties, 4 oz. 0
Turkey and corned beef:
(*Healthy Deli* Doubledecker), 1 oz. 0
Turkey frankfurter:
all varieties, 4 oz. 0
Turkey giblets or gizzards* 0
Turkey gravy:
canned (*Heinz* HomeStyle), ¼ cup 0
mix, prepared (*Lawry's*), 1 cup . . . . .2 c
Turkey ham:
all varieties, 4 oz. 0
Turkey luncheon meat:
all varieties, 4 oz. 0
Turkey pastrami:
all varieties, 4 oz. 0
Turkey salad spread:
(*Libby's Spreadables*), 1.9 oz. . . . . 1.0 d
Turkey salami:
all varieties, 4 oz. 0
Turkey sausage:
all varieties, 4 oz. 0
Turkey spread, canned:
chunky (*Underwood*), 1 oz. 0
Turkey summer sausage:
all varieties, 4 oz. 0
Turmeric, ground:
1 oz. . . . . 6.0 d
1 tsp. . . . . .5 d

Turnip, fresh or stored:

raw, without greens, untrimmed, 1 lb.	6.7 d
raw, trimmed, cubed, ½ cup	1.2 d
boiled, drained, cubed, ½ cup	1.6 d
boiled, drained, mashed, ½ cup	2.3 d

Turnip, frozen:

mashed, unheated, 3.3 oz.	1.7 d

Turnip greens, fresh:

raw, untrimmed, 1 lb.	7.6 d
raw, chopped, ½ cup	.7 d
boiled, drained, chopped, ½ cup	2.2 d

Turnip greens, canned:

with liquid, 4 oz.	1.5 d
with liquid, ½ cup	1.5 d
chopped, with diced turnips (Allens/Sunshine), ½ cup	1.0 d

Turnip greens, frozen, with turnips:

unheated, 3.3 oz.	2.3 d
boiled, drained, 4 oz.	3.5 d

V

Food and Measure	Fiber Grams

Vanilla extract:
(Virginia Dare), 1 tsp. 0
Veal* 0
Vegetable chow mein, canned:
meatless *(La Choy)*, ¾ cup . . . . 2.0 d
Vegetable juice cocktail, canned or bottled:
6 fl. oz. . . . . 1.0 d
all varieties *(R.W. Knudsen Very Veggie)*, 6 fl. oz. . 2.0 d
all varieties *("V-8")*, 6 fl. oz. . . . . 1.0 d
Vegetable oyster, see "Salsify"
Vegetable pocket sandwich, frozen:
Bar-B-Q *(Veggie Pockets)*, 5 oz. . . . . 1.5 d
broccoli cheddar *(Veggie Pockets)*, 5 oz. . . . . . . .2 d
Greek *(Veggie Pockets)*, 5 oz. . . . . <.1 d
Indian or Oriental *(Veggie Pockets)*, 5 oz. . . . . . . .9 d
pizza *(Veggie Pockets)*, 5 oz. . . . . 1.2 d
Tex-Mex *(Veggie Pockets)*, 5 oz. . . . . .3 d
Vegetable sticks, frozen:
(Stilwell), 5 pieces . . . . 2.0 d
Vegetable Stroganoff mix, prepared:
creamy *(Tofu Classics)*, ½ cup . . . . 1.9 d
Vegetables, see specific listings

Vegetables, mixed, canned:

with liquid[1], 4 oz. . . . . 4.3 d

with liquid[1], ½ cup . . . . 4.6 d

(Green Giant Garden Medley), ½ cup . . . . 1.0 d

(Green Giant Pantry Express), ½ cup . . . . 1.0 d

(La Choy Fancy Mix), ½ cup . . . . 1.0 d

chop suey *(La Choy),* ½ cup . . . . <1.0 d

Vegetables, mixed, frozen:

unheated[2], 4 oz. . . . . 5.1 d

boiled, drained[2], ½ cup . . . . 4.9 d

(Green Giant/Green Giant Harvest Fresh),

½ cup . . . . 2.0 d

for beef, Burgundy *(Birds Eye* Easy Recipe),

7 oz. . . . . 4.0 d

for beef, Italiano *(Birds Eye* Easy Recipe), 7 oz. . 3.0 d

in butter sauce *(Green Giant),* ½ cup . . . . 2.0 d

California or Western style *(Green Giant),*

½ cup . . . . 2.0 d

for chicken:

Alfredo *(Birds Eye* Easy Recipe), 7 oz. . . . . 3.0 d

glazed or teriyaki *(Birds Eye* Easy Recipe),

7 oz. . . . . 4.0 d

primavera *(Birds Eye* Easy Recipe), 7 oz. . . . . . 7.0 d

heartland style *(Green Giant),* ½ cup . . . . 2.5 d

Manhattan style *(Green Giant),* ½ cup . . . . 2.0 d

New England style *(Green Giant),* ½ cup . . . . . . 4.0 d

San Francisco, Santa Fe, or Seattle style

(Green Giant), ½ cup . . . . 2.5 d

Vegetarian burger, see " 'Hamburger,'

vegetarian"

Vegetarian chow mein mix:

Mandarin *(Tofu Classics),* prepared, ½ cup . . . . . 2.7 d

Venison* 0

---

[1] Includes carrots, green peas, green beans, and lima beans.

[2] Includes corn, lima beans, green beans, green peas, and carrots.

Vienna sausage, canned:

all varieties, 4 oz. 0

Vine spinach, raw:

untrimmed, 1 lb. . . . . 3.2 c

Vinegar:

all varieties 0

Vodka:

all varieties 0

W

Food and Measure	Fiber Grams

Waffle, frozen:

(Aunt Jemima Low Fat), 1 piece . . . . 4.7 d

(Eggo Nutri· Grain), 2 pieces . . . . 2.0 d

(Kellogg's Special K), 1 piece 0

plain or apple cinnamon (*Downyflake* Crisp &
   Healthy), 1 piece . . . . 1.0 d

plain or buttermilk, 1 piece, 4″ square,
   approximately 1.2 oz. . . . . .8 d

Belgian *(Belgian Chef),* 1 piece . . . . 6.0 d

multibran *(Eggo Nutri· Grain),* 2 pieces . . . . 5.0 d

oat bran *(Eggo),* 2 pieces . . . . 3.0 d

oat bran with fruit and nuts *(Eggo),* 2 pieces . . . . 4.0 d

raisin and bran *(Eggo Nutri· Grain),* 2 pieces . . . . 4.0 d

whole grain *(Roman Meal),* 1 piece . . . . 1.5 d

Waffle mix (see also "Pancake and waffle
   mix"), prepared:

complete, 1 piece, 7″ diameter, approximately
   2.6 oz. . . . . 1.1 d

complete, 1 piece, 9″ diameter, approximately
   7 oz. . . . . 2.8 d

Wakame, see "Seaweed"

Walnut oil:

all varieties 0

Walnut torte, see "Cake"

Walnuts, black, dried:

in shell, 1 lb. . . . .   5.4 d

shelled, 1 oz. . . . .   1.4 d

chopped, ½ cup . . . .   3.1 d

finely ground, ½ cup . . . .   2.0 d

Walnut, English or Persian, dried:

in shell, 1 lb. . . . .   9.8 d

shelled, 1 oz. . . . .   1.4 d

shelled, halves, ½ cup . . . .   2.4 d

pieces or chips, 1 cup . . . .   2.9 d

Water chestnuts (Chinese), fresh, raw:

untrimmed, 1 lb. . . . .   10.5 d

4 medium, 2″ diameter, approximately 1.3 oz. . . .   1.1 d

sliced, ½ cup . . . .   1.9 d

Water chestnuts, canned:

4 medium, approximately 1 oz. . . . .   .7 d

with liquid, 4 oz. . . . .   2.9 d

with liquid, sliced, ½ cup . . . .   1.8 d

(La Choy), 4 whole or ¼ cup sliced . . . .   <1.0 d

Watercress, fresh, raw:

untrimmed, 1 lb. . . . .   9.6 d

10 sprigs, 11¼″ long, approximately .9 oz. . . . . . .   .6 d

chopped, ½ cup . . . .   .4 d

Watermelon:

untrimmed, 1 lb. . . . .   1.2 d

1 slice, 1″ × 10″ diameter, approximately 2 lbs.

untrimmed . . . .   2.4 d

trimmed, diced, ½ cup . . . .   .4 d

Watermelon seeds, dried:

1 oz. . . . .   .9 c

Wax beans, see "Green beans"

Wax gourd:

raw:

untrimmed, 1 lb. . . . .   9.3 d

¼ gourd, approximately 4.4 lbs. untrimmed . . .   41.3 d

trimmed, cubed, ½ cup . . . .   1.9 d
boiled, drained, cubed, ½ cup . . . .   .9 d
Weakfish*   0
Wheat, whole grain:
hard red, spring or winter:
  2 oz. . . . .   7.1 d
  ½ cup . . . .   12.5 d
  (Arrowhead Mills), 2 oz. . . . .   8.3 d
soft red, for pastry *(Arrowhead Mills),* 2 oz. . . . . .   8.3 d
soft red, winter, 1 cup . . . .   2.9 c
Wheat, parboiled, see "Bulgur"
Wheat, sprouted:
1 oz. . . . .   .3 d
½ cup . . . .   .6 d
Wheat bran (see also "Cereal"), crude:
1 oz. . . . .   12.1 d
½ cup . . . .   12.7 d
2 tbsp. . . . .   3.0 d
(Kretschmer), 1 oz. or ⅓ cup . . . .   11.4 d
Wheat flakes:
(Arrowhead Mills), 2 oz. . . . .   6.7 d
Wheat flour:
pastry *(Arrowhead Mills),* 2 oz. . . . .   6.8 d
whole grain:
  2 oz. . . . .   6.9 d
  ½ cup . . . .   7.3 d
  (Pillsbury's Best), 1 cup . . . .   12.0 d
  stone ground *(Arrowhead Mills),* 2 oz. . . . .   6.7 d
white, all-purpose:
  2 oz. . . . .   1.9 d
  ½ cup . . . .   2.0 d
  (Ballard/Pillsbury's Best), 1 cup . . . .   2.0 d
  unbleached *(Pillsbury's Best),* 1 cup . . . .   3.0 d
white, bread:
  2 oz. . . . .   1.4 d

Wheat flour, white, bread *(cont.)*
½ cup . . . . 1.7 d
  (Pillsbury's Best), 1 cup . . . . 2.0 d
white, cake, 2 oz. . . . . 1.0 d
white, cake, ½ cup . . . . .9 d
white, self-rising:
  2 oz. . . . . 1.9 d
  ½ cup . . . . 2.0 d
  (Pillsbury's Best), 1 cup . . . . 2.0 d
Wheat germ:
(Kretschmer), 1 oz. . . . . 3.3 d
crude, 1 oz., approximately ¼ cup . . . . 3.7 d
crude, 2 tbsp. . . . . 1.9 d
honey crunch *(Kretschmer),* 1 oz. . . . . 3.0 d
raw *(Arrowhead Mills),* 2 oz. . . . . 6.5 d
toasted, 1 oz., approximately ¼ cup . . . . 3.7 d
toasted, 2 tbsp. . . . . 1.8 d
Wheat gluten:
(Arrowhead Mills Vital), 1 oz. . . . . .9 d
Wheat "nuts":
all flavors, unsalted, 1 oz. . . . . 1.5 d
Whelk* 0
Whey:
all varieties 0
Whipped topping:
dairy or nondairy 0
Whiskey:
all varieties 0
White bean and rice mix:
prepared *(Fantastic* Italiano), 10 oz. . . . . 8.0 d
White beans, dry:
uncooked, 1 oz. . . . . 4.3 d
boiled, ½ cup . . . . 5.7 d
small, boiled, ½ cup . . . . 3.7 d

White beans, canned:

with liquid, 4 oz. . . . . 5.5 d

with liquid, ½ cup . . . . 6.3 d

White Castle, 1 serving:

sandwiches:

   cheeseburger . . . . 2.7 d

   chicken . . . . 1.7 d

   fish, without tartar sauce . . . . 1.4 d

   hamburger . . . . 2.1 d

   sausage . . . . 2.0 d

   sausage with egg . . . . 3.0 d

side dishes:

   french fries . . . . 4.6 d

   onion chips . . . . 3.5 d

   onion rings . . . . 2.6 d

White sauce mix, dry:

1¾-oz. packet . . . . .1 c

Whitefish* 0

White-flowered gourd:

raw, untrimmed, 1 lb. . . . . 3.5 d

raw, 1 gourd, 17″ long, approximately 2.4 lbs.

   untrimmed . . . . 8.5 d

boiled, drained, 1″ cubes, ½ cup . . . . .5 c

Whiting* 0

Wieners:

meat or with cheese, 4 oz. 0

Wild rice:

uncooked, 1 oz. . . . . 1.8 d

uncooked, ½ cup . . . . 5.0 d

cooked:

   ½ cup . . . . 1.5 d

   (Fantastic Foods), ½ cup . . . . 2.0 d

   precooked *(Master Choice Texmati),* ½ cup . . . . .3 d

Wild rice mix, see "Rice dishes"

Wine:

all varieties 0

Wine cooler:
all varieties *(Bartles & Jaymes),* 6 fl. oz. 0
Winged beans, fresh:
raw, sliced, 1/2 cup . . . . .6 c
boiled, drained, 1/2 cup .4 c
Winged beans, dry:
raw, 1/2 cup . . . . 14.1 d
boiled, 1/2 cup . . . . 2.1 c
Winged bean leaves:
trimmed, 1 oz. . . . . .7 c
Winged bean tuber:
trimmed, 1 oz. . . . . 2.1 c
Winter squash (see also specific squash
  listings):
raw, untrimmed, 1 lb. 5.8 d
raw, trimmed, cubed, 1/2 cup . . . . 1.0 d
baked, cubed, 1/2 cup . . . . 2.9 d
Wolf fish* 0
Wonton wrapper:
1 piece, 31/2″ square 0
Worcestershire sauce:
(Heinz), 1 tbsp. 0
regular or white wine *(Lea & Perrins),* 1 tsp. 0
regular or hickory *(French's),* 1 tbsp. . . . . (0)

Y

Food and Measure	Fiber Grams

Yam:
raw, untrimmed, 1 lb. . . . . 16.0 d
raw, cubed, ½ cup . . . . 3.1 d
baked or boiled, cubed, ½ cup . . . . 2.7 d
Yam, canned or frozen, see "Sweet potato"
Yam, mountain, Hawaiian, see "Mountain
  yam"
Yam bean tuber, raw:
untrimmed, 1 lb. 20.5 d
1 slice, 4⅞" diameter × ⅛", approximately .2 oz.
  untrimmed . . . . .3 d
sliced, ½ cup . . . . 2.9 d
Yard-long beans, fresh:
boiled, drained, sliced, ½ cup . . . . .8 c
Yard-long beans, mature, dry:
raw, ½ cup . . . . 4.0 c
boiled, ½ cup . . . . 1.4 c
Yeast, baker's:
active, dry:
  ¼-oz. package . . . . 1.9 d
  1 tbsp. . . . . 3.3 d
  (Red Star), ¼ oz. . . . . 1.2 d
compressed, .6-oz. cake . . . . 1.6 d
Yellow beans, dry:
boiled, ½ cup . . . . 1.0 c

Yellow squash, see "Crookneck squash"
Yellow squash, frozen:
breaded *(Stilwell),* 6 pieces . . . .   1.0 d
Yellowtail*   0
Yogurt, regular:
plain, 8 oz. or 1 cup   0
fruit flavors, 8 oz. or 1 cup . . . .   (0)
Yogurt, frozen:
plain, 8 oz. or 1 cup   0
fruit flavors, 8 oz. or 1 cup . . . .   (0)
Yokan:
1 oz. . . . .   .4 c
1 slice, ¼″ thick, approximately ½ oz. . . . .   .2 c

Z

Food and Measure	Fiber Grams

Ziti, see "Pasta"
Zucchini, fresh, unpeeled:
raw:

untrimmed, 1 lb.	5.2 d
baby, 1 medium, 2⅝" long, approximately .4 oz. untrimmed	.2 d
baby, 1 large, 3⅛" long, approximately .6 oz. untrimmed	.3 d
trimmed, sliced, ½ cup	.8 d
boiled, drained, sliced, ½ cup	1.3 d
boiled, drained, mashed, ½ cup	1.7 d

Zucchini, canned:

Italian style *(Progresso)*, ½ cup	2.0 d
with tomato juice, ½ cup	.6 c

Zucchini, frozen, unpeeled:

unheated, 3.3 oz.	1.1 d

Zucchini sticks, frozen:

battered or breaded *(Stilwell)*, 8 sticks	2.0 d
breaded *(Quik-Krisp)*, 6 pieces	4.0 d

R for Good Health

from Bestselling Nutrition Expert
Lendon Smith, M.D.

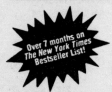

Over 7 months on
The New York Times
Bestseller List!

☐ **FEED YOUR KIDS RIGHT**
12706-8 $5.95

"Fascinating...a complete
nutritional program to ensure
a child's good health without
medicine."

—*American Baby* magazine

At your local bookstore or use this handy page for ordering:
DELL READERS SERVICE, DEPT. DLS
2451 South Wolf Road, Des Plaines, IL. 60018

Please send me the above title(s). I am enclosing $_____
(Please add $2.00 per order to cover shipping and handling.) Send
check or money order—no cash or C.O.D.s please.

Ms./Mrs./Mr. _____

Address _____

City/State _____ Zip _____
DLS-3/94

Prices and availability subject to change without notice. Please allow four to six
weeks for delivery.